Getting Joy in Your Life by Running

Strategies and Tips From 55 Years
To Enjoy Running and Life,
Whatever Your Age or Fitness Level,
While Slowing the
Deterioration of Your Body

Clifford Calderwood

RunToEnjoyLife.com

To: Ken,
Enjoy your Marathon
and Life!
Cliff Calder
10/1/2022

Getting Joy in Your Life by Running: Strategies and Tips From 55 Years to Enjoy Running and Life, Whatever Your Age or Fitness Level, While Slowing the Deterioration of Your Body

Clifford Calderwood

Copyright 2021 © Clifford Calderwood

Publisher: Ashumet Press

ISBN-13: 978-1-7372174-0-4

www.RunToEnjoyLife.com

Why Read This Book

At times it can seem all the running literature is reserved for only those serious about competition and winning ways. Still, we're all born runners, whatever our speed and commitment, and deserve more than a footnote covering the real reasons we run. More importantly, left unsaid are the lessons we can learn from our running that go far beyond just enjoying the next workout or race. Running can positively flavor our daily life with more enjoyment, but it requires a deliberate and authentic focus to enhance our thoughts and feelings to endure for life.

Whatever your athletic level and ambitions, and whether you've already run thousands of miles or are still looking to take your first running steps, this book is for you. It will:

- Reveal 10 strategies to enjoy and improve your running and life more.
- Open you to the art of listening to your body and mind to uncover the hidden lessons of running.
- Unleash the power of creativity and play into your workouts to stimulate your growth.
- Connect the importance and benefits of paying attention and avoiding distractions to relish your runs and reduce injuries.
- Disclose 5 running habits and their lessons to keep everything in your life in perspective.
- And much more…

With my young competitive racing days long over, I began a journey to understand how my running has helped me enjoy my life more and share it with others. So, tie up your laces, step outside, and get ready, because today is a good day for a good run, and this book is aimed at getting you more of those good days.

About the Author

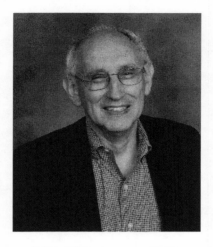

Clifford Calderwood is a lifelong runner. He was born and grew up in England, where he first fell under the spell of running as a young teenager. For the last 40 years, he's lived in Massachusetts, running its backroads, trails, hills, and beaches. Cliff has raced competitively on two continents and is an avid student of training schedules and techniques. In his journey of over five decades of running, he's studied what his relationship with his running activity is all about and why it's become necessary to his whole outlook on life.

Cliff is a retired Corporate IT Director and spent many years balancing the demands of work and personal life, including running. He's married with three sons and lives on Cape Cod, and has never really acclimatized to the New England winters but loves the diverse scenery of the Northeast.

Preface

I wrote this book during the COVID-19 pandemic. This is noteworthy because of the number of runners who communicated how running has helped get them through the isolation and confinement they felt during this period in our world history. When everything seemed in turmoil and unpredictable, there was their running to enjoy that provided a path not blocked, an activity not confined by the Coronavirus's events. This is the most significant endorsement of how the joy of running can impact our life.

We take much for granted during our time on Earth; freedom, family, friends, health, the sun continually rising, and the air we breathe to survive. When any of these are snatched from us, for whatever reason, suddenly we're reminded nothing is permanent and life is fragile.

So, there's no time to waste and only the present because yesterday is past and can't be changed, and tomorrow is only a promise and not guaranteed, but today is a good day for a good run.

East Falmouth
Massachusetts
May 2021

Disclaimer

Running is exercise, and you should use common sense when performing any exercise. If you've not exercised for an extended period or have been diagnosed with any heart condition, then it's recommended you have a discussion with your doctor and tell them your intent on running. Your doctor can determine any test to perform to expose any underlying issues you should be aware of before starting your running program.

Table of Contents

CHAPTER ONE

On your Marks...

"... Find out where joy resides and give it a voice far beyond singing. For to miss the joy is to miss all."
– Robert Louis Stevenson

I've been a lifelong runner.

I've run regularly to improve my running and stay healthy since my early teens. Apart from a few breaks, I've run consistently since the 1960s. I run because it's who I am and not just for the competition. I wasn't destined to become a champion athlete, but I was an above-average club runner in my youth and today remain competitive in my age group.

But my performance as a runner isn't the main story to share on these pages.

There's another side to running beyond the training and performance. Sure, running is all these if you desire, but it's much more. The discipline of running seeps into the veins of your life and changes other aspects beyond the role of fitness. Both running and its ability to influence your enjoyment of life is what I'll be exploring with you.

Running has had a significant impact on my life. Over the last 55+ years, I've amassed significant real-world experience in running, logged over 80,000 miles and still counting, and continue to enjoy a productive life into my seventies. I enjoy my running and life, and in these pages, I share my thoughts on both topics and how they can help you.

Any book like this is one person's perspective and opinions on the topic. All I ask of you is to try on what I share to see if it fits you. If it does, adopt it. If it doesn't, adjust and shape it until it does.

The running I'm going to be talking about isn't primarily about winning races or championships, although there are words for you here as well if you're on that journey. The approach I share is longer lasting than any schedule or single race, yet it's still about being the best you can be, whatever your current age or fitness level.

Some people make running complicated, a science to decipher, but it's simple. It's a natural movement we've done since we first stood upright. In the early days of our species, it helped save our life, and it still can if we learn how to surrender to its enchantment.

The running I'll be describing is a place of harmony and in the now, and where you're present all the time and are free to notice not only your running but also your surroundings. It may take some training, not only on how you run but also your mind, and more importantly, your thoughts. The fact is, when you run solo, you're doing all this anyway, but haphazardly. Why not regain control and let it inspire you beyond one run or only running but also in life?

Most people who run may not often think about its impact on them beyond a single session and how it can help them in their everyday lives. But to me, running is a metaphor for my life. When I run, its joy spills over into my other waking hours. The times in my life when I infrequently run, I "*missed*" it. Running is my therapy for sustained mental health.

It took me a long time to realize running is part of my identity, influencing my moods. I believe this is true for all of us who run, even if we're unaware of its underlying nature. I'll share what I discovered along my life journey through my running and how it has helped bring joy into my own life, and how it can do the same for you.

But first, a little of who I am and how I got here.

I started running as a high school sport, and I came to it with some natural ability. I grew up in England, where football is king and was my first love. I had better than average speed and skill and played soccer for my high school. But soccer is a fall and winter sport in the English school system. For the spring and summer months, there was only cricket and track and field for the boys. So, I focused on track and did well in the distance competition. My elder brother Richard ran competitively for the Royal Air Force, and watching some of his races inspired me to get more serious about my running. Richard was an excellent distance runner and possessed more natural speed than I. He introduced me to club running and a mentor—Johnny Walker— and eventually, I drifted into cross-country in the fall and winter months and road racing in spring and summer.

Road and cross-country races were my sweet spot. I'd train on grass tracks doing repetitions and on the streets and roads around where I lived in Sunbury-on-Thames. I had the most success racing through the fields and woods of southern England.

I enjoyed my early race successes running with Belgrave Harriers, a club located in Wimbledon, a suburb of London, more famous for the sport of tennis. I trained hard but in a few years reached a plateau and struggled to break through to the next level, no matter how many miles I ran in training or how many speed repetitions I did. My race performances were inconsistent, even if my training went well. It came to a point where I looked forward to workout but not racing competition, as it didn't give me the enjoyment or success I'd encountered earlier.

I've always enjoyed reading and learned all about the stars of that era through books and magazines. I read extensively about the era's track giants such as Ron Clark, Peter Snell, Murray Halberg, Jim Ryun, Herb Elliot, Michel Jazy, Kip Keino, Billy Mills, and Steve Prefontaine on the international front, and many English runners such as Bruce Tulloh, a young David Bedford, and later David Moorcroft, Steve Ovett, and Sebastian Coe. I studied their training methods, adapting a few to my capabilities, and followed the advice of various people who took me under their wing.

At that time, running for me was just a sport, and securing a career after leaving school soon became my focus. I also experienced some body chemistry changes that impacted my ability to enjoy my workouts, which stayed with me through my 20's. Eventually, due to these physical and emotional changes, my life's running went into hibernation and didn't fully wake up again until I moved to America.

It was in the early years of the 1980s when I got reacquainted with running. I'd moved to America for work and a thirst to see and experience more of the world, a travel trait I share with a number of my siblings. At the time, running was still enjoying its heyday, and my new company in Worcester, Massachusetts, had a vibrant lunchtime community of runners. Here also was an opportunity to meet people and enjoy my new life in a different country. I relished the community spirit of running again and found, though a little *"rusty,"* my running stamina, and some of my speed, hadn't deserted me entirely.

I also realized how much I missed running. Suddenly, I was back in my early days, following a consistent routine of running and enjoying myself. But it was different. I didn't have the pressures or expectations of youth or performance. I went out to run and not necessarily train for any event or race, although having a specific race goal helps keep me focused and out in all weathers. The fact was, I didn't run to be competitive with others but just to get outdoors and bathe in my therapy. I didn't realize this at the time or analyze it then but reflecting now, these were the running days where I formulated much of what I've learned about running and why it provides so much enjoyment to me.

Over the following decades, my running activities took a back seat again but never left entirely. I joined clubs such as Central Mass Striders in Worcester and today the Falmouth Running Club on Cape Cod, where I now live.

I juggled personal activities with helping to raise a family and having high-pressure jobs. But I would always, at some point, come back to my running. During these running droughts, I now realize there was some *"emptiness"* in my life, and the only way of filling it was to run. It wasn't an emptiness caused by unhappiness but just an enjoyment I'd once had that was now missing. Something that mainly became replaced by the joys of family life but not completely. Physical activity is in my DNA, and participating in sports has satisfied this need. I'm a runner.

Over the years, I reached a resolution with my running, understood how important it was to me, and realized it was part of who I was and how it made my life more enjoyable. It still does today. I found my enjoyment of life mirrored my level of happiness for my running.

It all starts with my running.

So, because I eventually understood this, I became careful and protective around my running and where it fitted in my life and attitude. Running for me is not just about health and fitness; it's a lens through which I see my life but not in an obsessive way.

I'm not trained in psychology and don't fully understand the therapeutic element of running in my life. I'm not always conscious of any psychology or physiological changes when running, especially on long runs of two hours. If there's a change, it begins the moment I step into my running shoes, like an actor stepping onto the stage. Will you experience this, or instead feel a difference further into your workout? I cannot say. I think it's different for each of us.

There are still days when running is a challenge for me. Life can be messy and unpredictable. My other commitments, the weather, my body, or my mood are all factors for me to get my run in for the day, as they'll be for you. Expect this and deal with it as best you can.

If you're familiar with and understand the term *"how you do anything is how you do everything,"* then you know this is all about mindset. Most people hear this saying first in a business setting, but it is also true in how you conduct your personal life. Make running significant in your life, then how you do it—your approach and philosophy around it—will spill over into the rest of your life and impact it. Your role is to ensure it's a positive impact and doesn't harm your enjoyment of life.

Remember, you're an individual with a unique experience in life. No one approach or schedule, or model will work for everybody. But that shouldn't stop you from being open to learning from others. Just be prepared to adapt and be flexible. You're shaped by your environment and experiences and will continue to be shaped by these, so make sure you choose wisely who and what to follow and be skeptical and discriminate. For, I've been there myself and felt good in the journey but empty at the destination.

My approach is slow and deliberate. There's no fast track to fitness and lasting joy, especially if you're not feeling it where you currently are. Instead, it's a way of thinking, so as you grow and change, you adapt your mindset as well. Some of my approaches may question icons you look up to now and want to imitate. It may make you doubt or rethink who you want to model. It may make you reevaluate the path of life you're on now. Be open to this, and you'll get the most out of this book.

By now, you've figured out I'm no spring chicken. I've been running now for over 5 decades and into my 6th since starting in my mid-teens. I intend to continue for as long as my body will let me. I have friends decades younger than me who can barely walk across the road. And yet, here I am, planning when to run my next 10K or marathon. I realize I'm fortunate. This book is not a training manual or schedule per se for elite or champion runners—although many have found their success in running hasn't spilled over into their personal life, so there is help here for them too—but it's more aimed at those of us who make up the remaining 99% of runners. Those of us who want to achieve a sustainable fitness level and help slow our body's deterioration, regardless of the state in which we approach this running journey. This book is for those who don't run just for the competition or the race but for the healthy joy and positive feelings it gives us.

In the final analysis, running is an individual activity. It's always a runner against themselves. At times it can feel lonely, but that does not mean you're alone. Millions are out there every day running. They're doing it for a multitude of reasons, each specific to their life and goals. When you meet another on the road, say hello or wave as you pass to acknowledge the fraternity you've joined.

In the following chapters, I'll share what I do today and what's working for me to keep my enjoyment of running into my seventies. I've condensed my approach down to 10 strategies. I think you'll be surprised at how simple and adaptable they are to make your own.

So, if you're ready to begin adding more enjoyment to your running and life, then let's move toward the starting line, and we'll begin our preparation with a few foundational elements.

On your marks...

CHAPTER TWO

Mindsets and Habits

"You have power over your mind — not outside events.
Realize this, and you will find strength."
— Marcus Aurelius

Whatever your reasons for joining me now in this journey, it doesn't matter; you'll get something out of this book. I promise to make our time together exciting and get you thinking about running in a different light.

But before we begin, there are a few important things I'd like you to know and understand before you slip into your sneakers and go out on your first or next run. Label these things what you will: *attitudes, mindsets, philosophies, habits,* or just *preparation.* It doesn't matter what you call each one as long as you let them enter your running mental repertoire. Whatever your experience with running or trepidations you may have about the enjoyment aspect of it, this time it'll be different if you include these aspects.

There is No Such Term as a Jogger:

The first is subtle, and you could say abstract. There's a difference between a jogging pace and a running pace, but it's relative to each runner. There is, however, no such term as a jogger; you're a runner. You may feel you're a slow runner initially, but in time this will change. So, please don't use the term jogger to describe to others, or yourself, your running activity. There's no rite of passage required before you can call yourself a runner. It's all how you think about it.

When I was a youth, I ran a 4:39 mile on a grass track barefoot. That was my fastest mile ever—I never bettered it. However, I would've been left in the dust and over 300 yards behind a four-minute miler in that race. But they wouldn't have run any harder or exerted more effort than I did. I lay flat-out exhausted at the end of the race, having, what seemed to me, sprinted for four laps. My point is, your running pace is all relative. You can expend as much effort running a 10-minute mile as another runner doing a 5-minute mile. You're no less a runner than them.

Even elite runners use the term jogging to mean an easy pace—for them. But their jogging pace for 10k could be my flat-out top speed for one mile.

So, when you put on your running shoes, adopt the mindset of being a runner, whatever your pace or fitness level. Don't slip into the comparison mode. Comparing your running abilities to others will ruin your enjoyment. There's no apology needed or feeling of embarrassment because of your size, style, or pace about calling yourself a runner. Remember that it works both ways when you whizz by somebody barely running faster than a walking pace and catch yourself thinking how slow they're going. The fact is, they're participating in an exercise activity that 99% of the population don't, so give them a wave of encouragement and respect.

We're born to run, and you're just exercising your heritage!

Style, Form, and Technique:

No, I'm not talking about the latest in shorts and tops that will turn heads next time you are out on the road or track—although there's nothing wrong with looking good when sweating profusely. The "*style*" I'm talking about is how you run and how it seems to others—coaches will call this technique or form. This style doesn't matter unless it's causing you physical discomfort or training for the shorter track events. How you run and where you hold your arms will fall to your physique and natural balance. I've read much about stride and upper body erectness and exactly where your arms should be when performing long-distance running, but there's little evidence it makes a difference.

I'm told my stride is too long and I run somewhat hunched over, which is all true. I've even been told I grimace a lot when running and look ready to collapse—in reality, I feel fine. If I seem a little flippant on this topic, it's because so much nonsense is written about it. Trying to change somebody's natural style is a devil of a job anyway. Even elite distance athletes have tried and given up.

The exceptions to my opinion above are if your technique is causing aches and pains to your body, or if you're a sprinter or in the 800/1500-meter events. My running style critique suggests I don't emulate a graceful gazelle when running, but it does not cause problems with my back or cause any other structural aches. If you suffer from these issues after a workout, seek professional advice, as your running style/form may be causing your problems.

Additionally, if you're training for any sprints or shorter track events, then style and form matter. To get the best performance for sprint events, learn how to use your arms, head, stride, and knee lift, which are critical to achieving peak performance. A qualified coach can help review what changes you need to make.

Goals for Motivation:

Have a goal for your running. Short term and long term if you want. I prefer to set a race goal. It is healthy and motivational to train for an event. It keeps the spark alive, particularly when the going gets tough or when weather or personal commitments cause friction in getting in a workout for the day. I cover this in more detail in a later chapter.

A word of caution on goals; be careful about tying your running to a weight goal. Running only for weight loss will likely be a disappointment to you. Running as the exercise, and to a degree, the emotional aspect of a weight maintenance program, makes sense. But other healthy habits, including nutrition and portion control, and your body chemistry, should be considered in reaching and maintaining your ideal weight.

Running Should be a Pleasant Tiredness:

The great New Zealand athletic coach, Arthur Lydiard, preached training to the point of pleasant tiredness. I like this thought, as it conveys a more realistic approach to running than the "*no pain no gain*" brigade of thinking, especially for those just beginning. Many people don't run or give up soon after starting, believing it to be too hard or painful. They see the grimaces on others out running and feel it will be painful and hurt them. Or they tried it once or twice, and they ached so much the next day they couldn't even put on their running gear. These attitudes or memories remain their backdrop and barrier to starting up or continuing.

Going into any exercise routine with the expectation it'll be challenging and will hurt; then, you've already conditioned your body through your mind to create this experience for you. So, instead, go in with the attitude it'll likely be uncomfortable at the beginning, like any exercise, but it shouldn't be hard at the initial stage. If it is, then you're doing too much too soon. A little self-regulation is needed out of the gate, and this includes not trying to run every day but taking rest days frequently. Even elite athletes schedule rest days or know when to take time off to recover.

While I talk about getting started in a later chapter, understand if you've been inactive for a while, then you need to acclimatize your body for running. The lower muscles and joints need to be conditioned, and by using some tender loving care while running, there's no reason to experience pain. This comes later... *just kidding*.

In the beginning, during your runs, you may feel uncomfortable and some stiffness the next day. In the first initial weeks, be gentle on your expectations and your body. Eventually, you'll need to push yourself if you want to improve on times and do longer runs. More on all this later.

Running and pain isn't an association I've experienced unless I'm injured. Either I can't run to or through pain, or my definition of "*pain*" is wildly different from others, I can't say because we can't experience what others feel. So, there's no need to expect running to be painful, nor should it be.

Some Days Running Just Sucks:

Another attitude essential for you is that one training run or race doesn't define your running relationship. You're the sum of all your life so far and not one event or activity. The great Australian runner, Ron Clarke, never won an Olympic Gold Medal. However, his work body, including a phenomenal period of consistently breaking world records, is still admired today by runners of all ages. His book *The Unforgiving Minute* details all his major races and echoes a lot of what I am saying. It's worth a read.

You'll have training runs when you suck—physically as well as mentally. The same will be true of a race you may enter. Despite all the excellent preparation and great times during training sessions on race day, it can all fall apart and be a major disappointment to you. But you're not a machine or a tap to turn on and off and expect it to work each time flawlessly.

In preparation for one of my marathons, I obtained and slightly adapted a schedule for my training and faithfully followed it. Training mostly went well over the 16-weeks, and I approached the race well-prepared and with a positive attitude. The race day weather wasn't great, and I had a disappointing run and finished 35 minutes off my target time. I just didn't have it that day—no excuses. I rested for one week and then was planning my next marathon.

Just like life, running can be unpredictable as well.

Keep a Mileage Logbook:

Get into the habit of keeping a simple logbook of your mileage. I'm not one to document details about my sessions or how I felt, just the facts. How many miles I did, my time, and notes on weather conditions. I use a page a week. But of course, you can capture all manner of things about your training sessions—it could be a sort of memoir if you wish but entirely your choice.

But the essential miles covered and the time it takes will provide you all the data you'll need, and it'll help motivate you as you see your mileage increase and your times decrease. I'll explain in subsequent chapters how you can use the information you collect to make decisions about equipment and races. There's no need to buy expensive journals—a cheap spiral-bound 200-page notebook will last for four years or longer.

Make Running Playful:

Make your running sessions fun. Now, I'm not suggesting you don't treat your time exercising seriously to get the results you want, but so many people quickly get bored with the same route, schedule, and pace. Just as in life, we need to sprinkle some fun over our leisure activities. I've some ways of spicing your sessions up for you and making your running fun while keeping on target. But just understand there's nothing wrong with mixing playtime with your exercise routine.

Conversations with your Physician:

Before starting any vigorous physical program such as running, you should discuss with your physician your intent on running and if a stress test is required. The stress test will provide you with information about your heart and its ability to support strenuous exercise and your maximum and target heart rate. As a runner, you should know and understand heart rates and monitor them both at rest and during exercise.

Running is primarily aerobic exercise, and your heart will love you for keeping it healthy this way. But you should know the current health of your heart and its capabilities before starting your program. Medical doctors come in all shapes and sizes, and some of them are runners. If possible, choose a physician who runs, as this will give you confidence in the information you're getting from their personal experience.

So, I've introduced you to some mindsets and attitudes and habits of approaching your running, and now it's time to introduce you to the ten strategies for getting more joy out of your life by running. The next chapter will run you through a summary of all ten, and then I'll dive deeper into each one in the following chapters of the book.

CHAPTER THREE

On the 10 Ways to Enjoy
Your Running and Life

"I Don't run to add days to my life,
I run to add life to my days."
— Ronald Rook

S o, you're probably wondering what exactly I will be sharing with you that you haven't heard already? What *"secrets"* lie in these pages that'll suddenly make your running and life different?

You're going to have to do *"work"* and get sweaty and experiment, and it'll require a hefty dose of self-motivation. There are no shortcuts, but there are many long detours and distractions you can avoid. I'll do my best to point these out as we take this journey together.

I'll discuss many aspects of running and related topics based on my decades of real-world experiences. Over the years, I've also studied famous athletes, world-renowned coaches and implemented a library of training schedules and workout regimes. You'll get the most out of your reading if you keep an open and curious mind and continually ask yourself, *"what does this mean for me?"*

You may disagree or not relate to some of the approaches and mindsets I share with you. That's fine by me. However, just because your experience differs significantly from mine in some respects, don't fall into the trap of *'throwing the baby out with the bathwater."* This, after all, is a common reason why we get stuck in life and don't change. I wish I'd a penny for everybody who has said to me *"but I know all this because I've heard it before..."* So, what did you do with the knowledge you already had? Timing is everything. Rehearing something again at a different time in your life when it's suddenly relevant can give you the nudge you need now to make a massive difference in your running and life.

Think then of the following as a quick summary of the next ten chapters on the ten strategies I'll be sharing.

Listening to your Body and Mind:

We've much to learn from others if we but listen and absorb without prejudice. This isn't as easy as it may sound, as each day we come to our life's table with years of being shaped by our environment and experiences. It can be a devil to leave our proverbial *"life's coat at the door"* as we step through the entrance into another day. After all, it's a chance to gain new insights into ourselves and begin to unravel and replace the clothing that isn't beneficially serving us any longer.

Listening then is no less a skill than talking. It's said you should spend two-thirds listening and one-third talking. It's then essential we agree to pay attention to our thoughts. After all, you do hear all your thoughts, but you're not listening to them most of the time. It does take effort and practice, but the rewards will be immense if you want to change.

While I talk about it in the context of running and how it'll help you enjoy exercise more and protect you from injury, you'll also discover how it can help you shape your happiness in life.

Major and Minor Props:

Running isn't an expensive activity. The most crucial piece of equipment you need to run is a quality pair of running shoes. It's obvious, I know, but what you put on your feet provides the principal protection between your body and the surface you run on. Your shoes must also be replaced regularly, likely a lot sooner than you would expect and prefer, given the cost for a quality pair.

Depending on your location's climate, other significant equipment to purchase is anything to keep you warm, protected, and comfortable, such as leggings, tops, gloves, socks, and hats—shop discount for this stuff.

Then comes a whole array of "*nice to have*" equipment that I class as minor props and depends on your budget. I liken these props to what you may surround yourself with in your life to make it more pleasant and generally are *wants* rather than *needs*.

The Power of Play:

Your running should be fun. You should look forward to it and anticipate getting absorbed and "*lost*" mentally in your training runs. It shouldn't turn into a chore, seem like work, or make you feel guilty or selfish. Consider it an opportunity to play as you did when you were a kid.

You can achieve this playfulness by spicing up your training runs. Examples of keeping up the interest include introducing fartlek training, mixing different paces throughout the session, trying different routes or environments to run in, and more.

We can get stuck in our routines and forget our reasons for starting an activity in the first place. This can happen in our lives if we don't pay attention, and one day we wake up and wonder how we got to where we are.

Paying Attention and Avoiding Distractions:

You'll find I'm an advocate of running outdoors as long as it isn't hazardous for your health or safety. I feel we've lost the art of enjoying the outdoors and nature. For the most part, we don't pay attention to the environment when outside—we take it for granted or ignore it completely. We instead look for distractions such as running with earbuds swamped in music or listening to self-improvement programs as we pound the pavement. It's as if the activity and the outdoors aren't enjoyable enough to hold our attention. I've even seen people running answering a phone call—what's that all about? Adding any distraction to our restoration periods seems to defeat the whole premise of time to refresh.

Not paying attention when running is both a wasted opportunity to enjoy the outdoors and detrimental to our safety and health. It can cause injuries and accidents, many of which can be avoided.

Rainy Mornings and Sunny Afternoons:

There's no one ideal time to run for the day; at least, I've never found one. No science proves running first thing in the morning is best, or at lunchtime or in the evening. You decide on your daily routine and what works best for you. I've found though my running allows me to hit my refresh button on the day. A *"bad"* morning when the mood is low or unexpected problems appear and seem to accumulate can take on a different perspective after a run.

A run for the day also provides the opportunity to work problems through during the enjoyment of exercise. This isn't at odds with my thoughts on distractions as it's channeling attention to a specific issue "*on your mind*" anyway. The detail in this chapter will take you through different scenarios on turning a "*rainy day*" into a "*sunny day*" through your running, regardless of where in the day you fit it in.

Reducing and Recovering from Injuries:

I've been injured in my running life, a few injuries kept me out for weeks, but only one turned into months. Compared to many who run, it's been a small number and never to a point where I've felt I need to give up running and do some other sport. I can count on one hand the injuries that have kept me from running for more than a week. My running has also helped keep my joints free of aches and still does to this day. I'll share some guidelines I use to reduce the number of injuries my running has introduced.

The section on recovering from injuries is purely down to my experience in getting back to running when an injury occurs. For a runner, the recuperation period is frustrating. Still, there are ways to minimize the damage when accidents happen, helping to shorten any injury time and nursing your leg joints and muscles back to health.

Avoiding "Burnout" But Keeping the Edge:

Burnout happens when we put our body under stress for an extended period. In our running, this can be caused by having repeated hard training sessions and not allowing our bodies time to recover. If you're an elite or champion runner, then punishing your body on an almost daily basis can leave you with nothing to give in a competitive race.

For the leisure runner, it's a simple trap to tackle too much too soon, especially if you've got a competitive personality. There's nothing unhealthy in this, and indeed the stress you put your body under in your training sessions and how often to do this is your choice. But there's a balance to be found in avoiding burnout in your running yet keeping an edge to your training sessions to meet whatever goals you have set but still enjoy the journey.

If your goal is focused on a specific race, then ensuring you're ready to perform at your best for it requires achieving that balance, lest you find your best run is left on the "*road*" or "*track*" in your training sessions. In this chapter, I discuss ways to achieve balance for your running and life.

Fuel for Your Body:

If you want to be healthy and fit, and one way of measuring this is our body's resistance to disease and illness, then it's universal knowledge you must be careful of what foods you put in your body to fuel it. It'll be of no surprise to you that our life expectancy can be severely hampered by eating or drinking "*bad*" fuel. I'm not a nutritionist or against alcohol, but I've seen the cause and effect of people consuming a diet of food and drink that kills them early in their life. But this chapter isn't about what specific foods you should eat—likely you know this already—but more about how to navigate through the food and drink minefield, making sure you feed your running and life with predominately nutritious food and reasonable portion sizes.

If you want to be the best you can be in your running and life, then paying attention and listening to your body regarding the fuel you place in it plays a critical part. It does come down to common sense and habits, and I'll share what has helped me keep to a principal balance of healthy food and drink intake.

Mapping Out Your World:

Common threads in my attitudes and realistic practicalities toward running are a careful choice of routes, plenty of diversity, planning a weekly schedule, and the importance of scheduling rest days. There's an interplay in all these and their impact on your enjoyment, safety, and performance. As I talked about keeping the *"edge"* in your running previously, this chapter is about keeping the *"spark."*

Setting expectations for your running that test your limits is healthy. Probing your capabilities will increase your stamina and speed. You'll find improvements will come gradually and even in plateau levels. During this time, it's easy to become stale. The same routine, same route, same pace, and everything can quickly make life feel dull.

So, I'll share thoughts on mapping out a world for you to keep the enjoyment omnipresent.

Keeping Everything in Perspective:

Running is an activity I love to do, and it's part of my identity, but it's not my whole life. In my early days, when I was a competitive racer, it was more important than now. Depending on your goals and where you are in your life, you'll decide the importance it'll play. There's no right or wrong to this if you keep it healthy and in perspective with the rest of your life activities.

I grew up in a close family, and we're still close and communicate regularly. I've got a wonderful wife and three marvelous sons, as well as a brother and two sisters in the UK. Outside my running, I've other goals and activities that take my time. I'm grateful for running and the lessons it has taught me for life. It took me decades to discover how to leverage these lessons, and I share my journey in this chapter and hope it helps you keep whatever perspective makes sense for you.

I've created two closing chapters after the strategy chapters. I believe there's always value in integrating the salient points and a sense of what can come next after you finish and put any non-fiction book down. And so, in the final chapters, I'll cover how I've tied together in my life what I've learned from my running as an example for you and how you can use it your own and go beyond.

We've arrived at the place to begin the details, and we start with the real art of listening to your body and mind and the many ways it can benefit you.

It's time to step outside to prepare and explore...

CHAPTER FOUR

Listening to Your Body and Mind

Mens sana in corpore sano –
"A healthy mind in a healthy body."

Pain is your body's way of telling you something is wrong. It's a sign something is going on, needing your attention.

There are different kinds of hurt, and the two obvious ones are physical and emotional. I'll start with physical pain and discomfort. The type where you'll check things out where the pain is coming from to identify the source. Later on, I'll cover emotional pain.

The cause of physical pain may be apparent such as a cut or bruise you can see and attend to. Other times it's internal, and you know the general region but cannot see visible signs of the cause. Depending on the intensity and what we can see physically, we urgently attend to it—think ER at a hospital—or schedule a doctor visit.

The point here is we're "**listening to our body**." We're paying attention to whatever may be causing us pain.

You can get all kinds of soreness that crop up while running. There are what runners call spasms, and of course, a runner's stitch. None of these usually require drastic action; a typical response is running through it or stopping for a few minutes and waiting until it subsides. I get twinges all the time. I usually run through them unless it persists and causes me to change my stride or gate, and then I stop and maybe walk it off. A runner's or side stitch, for me, tends to happen in a race but can happen in a workout run. These stitches and twinges are harmless and usually disappear within a few minutes.

The point in all this is that listening to your body is natural, and we do it all the time, but it's usually triggered by a feeling something isn't right, which can happen during any run. We can suddenly be conscious of pain or discomfort that was not there before and act upon it. But there is value in, as part of our warmup routine, deliberately thinking about how we're feeling. You ask, essentially, if your body is prepared to run today? Is it ready to support you in what you've scheduled or planned for your workout today?

They're simple questions, and you listen for the answer. And you pay attention and act on it. Listening to your body then includes listening to how you feel. At this point, I'm still referring to how you feel physically.

I know my body (and my risk factor) well enough that physical tiredness is a threat to me. I submit it's a threat to any runner. When you're tired, especially in your legs, having a nagging soreness or stiffness, then this can be a recipe for disaster. This is when missteps and mistakes can cause injuries, especially when running outdoors on the road.

Doing a long run or an intense track session can cause tiredness the next day. I anticipate this now and tend to schedule a rest day after a long run or an exceptionally long or hard-speed session. If the run was particularly long for me—10 – 12 miles, but sometimes when preparing for a marathon, it can be 18 – 20 miles—then it may take me multiple days to recover. And on the third day, it may be an easy run day, a short distance, and a slow pace.

After my last marathon, I rested my body for one whole week and was not back into any consistent schedule for another week. The body needs time to recover from such a demand, and the marathon can cause a mental and physical drain.

To the younger elite and champion runner, dealing with tiredness or soreness by resting this way can sound like a missed opportunity to toughen up. A time when you should be pushing through and training your body to increase stamina to accept tiredness and discomfort and continue +on. A time not to rest but to train your body to endure through duress and prepare better for the hurt of a race. I understand, and I had those days as well once. But I'm also talking to the beginner or runner who wishes to approach their running capabilities with less urgency and risk.

I've had running sessions where I felt okay starting, but after less than a mile, I knew I was in trouble, and it was going to be a hard slog to get through what I'd planned. Ignoring what my body was telling me wasn't in my best interest. I've had days where I knew almost immediately to turn around and get back home. In some rare instances, walk, not run, home. Preserve me for another day. There are days when it benefits your body to have an unscheduled rest day and substitute with a walk or other exercise type.

I'm describing a different way of listening to your body but every bit as necessary. It's a way of making sure you keep enjoying your running. Running should be a joy to feel the freedom of the outside and participate in the exercise. You release chemicals when running that can give you a euphoric feeling. There's also a sense of purpose when you complete your run and reach a target.

But there are times when you should save yourself for another day. There's always tomorrow.

There's another type of listening to your body that, for runners, is equally important. And that's how your body is feeling emotionally on the day. We've got an expression for this in England—are you feeling "*out of sorts*?" This means you don't feel 100 percent okay for whatever reason.

You see, where it becomes more challenging to listen is when there's no pain or discomfort or twinges, but you're tired or feel drained and ignore these signs because, well, it's not uncomfortable to run. If you feel emotionally drained because of something going on in your life, getting out for a run may be the best thing to rekindle your spirits.

Here, I want to talk about emotional tiredness or hurt, for it happens to all of us. It can be just as dangerous because it can cause injuries due to the distraction it can have on us. But running can also be an excellent antidote for this kind of tiredness. We can't have a great day every day. Some days we feel all is right with the world, and other days it can be tough to get through. We tell ourselves we should have stayed in bed; things are not going well for us. It may seem everything we touch or attempt to do seems to go wrong. Life can be messy.

Running can be our therapy to help us through these days.

This is an excellent place to highlight more about running as therapy, and there are several books that explore in detail the use of this as a therapy. They talk about running to recover from a significant illness to severe depression. These books cover studies and research from medical doctors and those more qualified than I to represent the benefits. Though I've read a selection of these books, up to now in my life, I've not personally had any significant illnesses or suffered from severe depression. I can only relate to my own experiences regarding running as therapy, and it's been extremely positive for me.

John Ratey, MD, has written a seminal work on exercise to treat mental health issues and laments that the overall medical professions continue to focus on medications and little endorsement of exercise as a treatment. His book *Spark: The Revolutionary New Science of Exercise and the Brain* is worth reading. It provides the science behind why your body and mind benefit from it, regardless of whether you suffer from anxiety and depression.

When the sky is cloudy and rainy, both actual and metaphorically speaking, and our mood is dark and low, running can help us get to a better place. For me, this is a quick and straightforward process to achieve a better state of wellbeing. But for others reading this, I realize it can be complicated and take longer, and the books covering this topic can provide further insight and guidance for you. I mention a few in the bibliography section and more at the companion website www.RunToEnjoyLife.com

But even in my life, running isn't always the best therapy. If the way I feel on any day will put me at risk by running rather than helping me, I listen to my body and mind and pass on running that day. I may go for a long walk or do something else I enjoy doing, such as drawing—it's always good to have another activity you enjoy when you cannot or shouldn't run.

If, however, I feel running that day is needed to help me out of a slump, then I'm anxious to get going. There is, after all, a real chance somewhere during the run I'll get absorbed in being outside and enjoy the therapeutic process. I'm generally a positive person, an optimist as they say, and I invariably see my glass always half full. But I'm not a slave to running, and I can skip a running day without feeling guilty.

But I realize everybody is different, and there should be no negative judgment on coming to a different conclusion in determining if you should run that day.

Is this a slippery slope?

It can be. We make up all kinds of stories for not doing something. We're good at that. I can do this in many areas of my life... but not running. You see, we don't tend to do this on things we enjoy doing. I've other areas of my life where I'm not so consistent and procrastinate easier and give myself opportunities to delay attending a decision or chore. We all have these things or activities in our life. I'm no different.

But not when it comes to running. And here is the thing, running provides me the thinking vehicle that gets me in the mood to tackle those things I'm putting off. It helps me put them in perspective and identify when my mind is tricking me into, or out of, an action or decision, and once exposed, I can make a different choice.

Wow, all that from just running, you ask?

Yes, for me. This is one of those occasions when running, even when I may not feel 100% ready or in the spirit, helps me get through a difficult time and back to enjoying life. Because likely you've noticed when you feel low or are just having a tough emotional day, then it's about everything in your life at that time. It seems all around is falling apart for you, and if these are your thoughts, they lead to you feeling that way.

Your thoughts lead to your feelings. So, controlling your thoughts becomes a critical element in how you feel about your running and life. Most of us are excellent at listening to the thoughts in our mind when they're negative or don't fit with our opinions or view of the world. This isn't the time to explore this rabbit hole further, but I'll share some further reading in the bibliography section around "*The Three Principles*" framework developed by Sydney Banks. You'll find this enlightening in increasing your joy in life.

Running then can help you break out of those negative thoughts and feelings. This is a different type of listening and is about listening to your mind.

Listening to your body and feelings can take practice. As I discussed, in some instances, it's about concluding to take a rest day or ease off on a challenging or intense training session. It is about reducing the risk of injury. It's not about avoidance because of laziness or being soft. It's a positive decision aimed at protecting your body. In other instances, it's about deciding to forge ahead regardless because you need the therapy of running to help overcome a day that will remain dark even if you choose to skip your run for the day.

You get to decide based on your experience of yourself and your body and its needs that day. So, be mindful of this. Live in the present as our mindfulness colleagues and teachers tell us.

It took me a long time to realize and understand the importance of running to me and its impact on my life enjoyment. I started running seriously at a young age because I'd some natural ability that also provided joy that I derived from it. Then it became a way of keeping fit and staying healthy. Eventually, it became part of my identity, and I missed it if I didn't do it. So, I always came back to it, even after spells of neglect. It took me a while to appreciate that running was essential to me and that not running for long periods was detrimental to my wellbeing and enjoyment of life.

You could say it took me a while to listen to my body and mind and the importance of running in keeping it in balance. There's no reason why it should take you as long as it took me to discover this. There's every reason why regardless of how you feel about running today, it can become a source of enjoyment to you and be able to take those feelings into other aspects of your life.

Become an excellent listener, as it's one of the most important gifts you can give yourself. It helps us be better people for others, but just as importantly, for ourselves.

So, after all this "*listening,*" you're good to put on your shoes, shorts, and a top and get out to the park or roads, right? Hang on there. Before you do, it's time to discuss your gear, and one especially critical piece you shouldn't take a single running step before you get right. I'll cover this and other major and minor props you should be purchasing in the next chapter.

CHAPTER FIVE

Major and Minor Props

*"Comfortable shoes and the freedom to leave are
the two most important things in life"*
— Shel Silverstein

R unning isn't inherently an expensive activity to participate
in. Put on a pair of sneakers, socks, shorts, and a top lying
around, and you're good to go and run outside. No
expensive gym membership is required. The last time I checked,
running on streets, roads, or a high school track was still free.

Of course, climate can affect your costs. Northern climates in
the winter demand more clothing to keep you warm outside. Yes,
I live in a cold winter climate, and running year-round in New
England presents some gear planning and costs. You'll see how
I thrive without breaking the bank in this chapter.

When it comes to running, the most crucial equipment in your
armory is your shoes. This is literally where the *"rubber"* meets
the road and where you should invest most of your dollars and
not skimp. You can be a cheapskate on shorts and tops and even

socks for clothing, but when it comes to what you put on the sole of your feet, you must spend the money to get the best support for your body to replace them frequently.

Yes, the running shoe companies have indeed developed all types of gimmicks to get you to part with your hard-earned money, so become an educated buyer. Understand your requirements in a shoe, do the research and read reviews.

The type of running shoes you purchase should be chosen carefully, and the first time should be done with the help of a store assistant who's also a runner. It's a specialized industry. Choosing the correct pair for you shouldn't only consider your foot size but the support you need and your gait.

I don't order shoes through online stores. Shoes, to me, are something you try on in a store and walk up and down and get a feel for them. Do they pinch? Do I need a wide fit in this model? Is there some wiggle room at the front of the shoe? What size for this manufacturer works best for me? Do they compensate for my running gait—the way my feet hit the ground with each stride—Do I pronate when I run? Will this shoe make me pronate more? Do they give my leg bones, joints, and muscles the support I need?

This may seem like many questions to get answered, but each one is critical to your comfort and avoiding injuries.

Insufficient support in your running shoe increases the risk of injuries. When you run, there's a tremendous force hitting the ground with each impact of your stride. Reducing the impact by having excellent support for your legs and body is critical.

In the early days of my running, there was little attention paid to support in the shoes. Lightness was considered king for training and race shoes. Today, the advancement has produced bulky shock absorbers for the feet, using materials chosen for their strength and light weight. An excellent pair of running shoes should give you great support for your training and races. Again, I urge you not to pop into a local department store sneaker section and pick up a pair of discounted shoes.

Find a manufacturer and model that provides you the cushioning you like and stick with them. Your leg muscles generally compensate for different cushioning, although too thin should be avoided. Manufacturers upgrade their models regularly as they look to provide more support for the same price by producing a shoe using the latest in design and materials. But the proof is in the individual experience you get with a pair. While it may be boring to keep buying the same shoes, there's protection in knowing what you're getting.

The other noteworthy discussion about running shoes is how long do they last? For many distance runners, just a few months' wear is all they get out of them. Running on them compresses the cushioning support over time, a relatively short time compared to a pair of walking sneakers or dress shoes. For the cynic, the self-serving recommended mileage for a pair of running shoes is anywhere from 250–500 miles. I find I can get at least 750 miles out of my shoes before I begin to see and "*feel*" the breakdown. A visible inspection of the shoe's sole will show the wear, particularly on the heel area. The shoe should show consistent wear on either side. If one side is worn further down, then this is evidence of pronation, and you should discuss this with your coach or someone qualified and you trust.

This is another one of those "*listen to your body*" moments. I tend to feel it first in my knees, and this happens anywhere between 500-750 miles for me.

Champion athletes will lean on the low side and change more frequently, but many are sponsored and don't pay for their shoes. Likely, you're not an elite runner, and so the cost does matter to you.

So, you'll need to keep a running log of your miles on each different shoe you use—some runners (not me) have multiple shoes and alternate. This is important. I keep a weekly log per page and just put down the mileage each day and my time and tally it up at the end of the week. A cheap small notebook works for me. It lasts for a few years but provides a minimal record of my training and mileage. I don't record like a journal describing how I felt, etc. But some people do, and if this works for you, go for it.

The fact is, depending on how many miles you run weekly, then you'll be changing your shoes every 4-6 months. If you're starting and easing into running, you'll likely get a long time out of your shoes. Ten miles a week will push you closer to a year out of your shoes, and this is fine if you use your shoes only for running.

Outside running shoes, then everything else is primarily optional and your preference.

I prefer to wear ankle socks in my shoes. I like something between my bare feet and the inner shoe. It stops me from getting blisters and other sores and reduces sweat in the shoe. It doesn't protect my toenails, and I still lose the occasional big toenail over time. A poorly fitting shoe can be a culprit in blackened toenails, but in my case, I don't feel it has anything to do with my shoe fittings.

I prefer any material that can absorb my sweat when it comes to shorts and tops, but I've not found anything for the running I do that's worth spending a lot of money on to get better absorption and comfort. As an older male, any top can cause friction on my nipples and cause bleeding. I have tried nipple guards, but they're an expensive solution, and frankly, I've never been able to make them stick consistently. For me, Vaseline works better and is cheaper but over time soils your tops. I also find Vaseline can be used for other areas that rub against clothing and the inside of my groin.

As an aside, I feel most information I've included in this book so far has been gender-neutral. However, I recognize that females will have specific requirements for sportswear, and aside from the fact that women will want support for their breasts and comfort, men will need support for their testicles. I prefer shorts with an inside lining rather than a separate strap or briefs. I think those are the primary differences in gear I need to mention.

I tend to buy socks, shorts, and tops in bulk online and have found a manufacturer whose products I prefer, and that's a reasonable price. Don't get hung up on clothing but focus on being comfortable. Once again, save the bulk of your budget for your shoes.

As I live in New England, our winters can be harsh. Running in below-freezing temperatures in the cold months is typical. I avoid running outside when the mercury falls below 12F for safety and comfort because I like to be warm to enjoy my running. Even on cooler rainy days of spring or fall, I wear a hat and gloves that keep these extremities protected and warm. I also have fleece balaclava ski masks that keep the cold wind off my face, but I don't find too many days when they're needed living near the ocean.

In the cooler months and through winter, I wear thermal cyclist tights. I prefer these to regular training pants. I like their snugness, and they keep me plenty warm even in the coldest temperatures. I wear shorts over them, ala Superman-style—but there the resemblance to the superhero ends, folks!

My weak points are my hands. Special running gloves that keep fingers warm in freezing temperatures are expensive. Anywhere from $45-$60 per pair. I've not found they offer warmer protection than a cheaper pair of regular fleece-lined gloves. The main selling point of running gloves is they're designed so you can still operate any electronic equipment you take out with you without taking the gloves off. I've not found these to be worth the cost, but you may feel differently. I have a few pairs of running gloves, which I reuse during the week before washing. Gloves do pick up a sweat, but I find they keep my hands warm for multiple sessions after drying out. I don't see even in the Northeast a need for hand warmers in the winter. One of my hands tends to get colder quicker than the other. As you get older, circulation becomes a factor, and sometimes there doesn't seem any rhyme or reason for what gets cold first.

I don't like being cold when running, so I also wear a hat in cooler weather. I find running caps are not expensive, but you may not need them. I have winter tops I use that have hoods, but I prefer a hat for my head or my balaclavas for extreme conditions. I have a small head and find the hood on the top flaps around and annoys me when I'm running. The winter tops I purchase have the thickness I prefer but only come with a hood, so I tuck the hood inside when wearing it, so it doesn't flap around.

I also wear long socks in the winter, but this is more to limit my skin to exposure and help me through the initial few miles when my body is still adjusting to the elements. I don't find I need extra thickness in my socks in the winter for warmth. The action of running is naturally pumping extra blood through my feet and keeping them warm.

So, where does technology come into all this running gear? Not a lot. It comes down to what you find helpful, wants, and are prepared to pay to get.

Before the advent of GPS in a watch, I'd get familiar with my routes and their length and mileposts by driving them, looking at the odometer, and matching them with landmarks such as specific trees or house or lamp posts. Knowing the mile markers would give me everything I needed to know to perform my short and long runs, confirm my pace and do any fartlek/speed workouts.

This is still good enough for most folks. After all, when starting, it's more important you run for time than mileage. But you should have a good approximate for tracking your mileage each session, even if you only need it for knowing when to replace your shoes.

My only real piece of technology luxury when it comes to running is my watch. These days I like to be able to track my mileage without mentally keeping track of it. I've got a watch with GPS, and it tracks my pace and mileage. It has all kinds of nifty programs on it, and if I'd the inclination to read the detailed instructions, I could engage it more to manage my fartlek/speed training, but I don't. I keep it simple. I live in a rural area, and it seems it takes a while to find the satellites, but it always does eventually. So, I switch it to this mode when doing my stretching exercises, and by the time I've finished stretching, it beeps to let me know it's ready to start and track my running.

I do find these watches only provide approximate details. Depending on the time I perform my run, the mileage may vary slightly from workout to workout, even if the route is the same. It's not a large discrepancy but just something to keep in mind, especially when using it for fartlek session tracking.

My watch also has an indoor mode to track my mileage when I'm forced to run on the treadmill, but frankly, in this mode, it's even less accurate and not to be trusted, and I prefer to rely on my treadmill mechanism knowing that's not precise either.

So, these watches aren't perfect, but I like my watch, and it looks good and small enough to keep on my wrist all day and night— it tracks my sleep time and heart rate. Both are useful for me to know at my age, and it's appropriate to confirm my average resting heart rate—more about this in my habits section in chapter 12. The watch cost me $100 when new, but I've had it for a few years now, so it keeps on giving. I just need to keep an eye out when it needs charging—usually once or twice a week.

For those who want to monitor their target heart rate during running as part of a program or keep within a range and don't exceed it, this alone may be worth investing in one of these gadgets. Sure, you can take your pulse with your fingers, but good luck with doing that during a training session.

There are watches on the market where you can download music or other MP3 files. Still, I have strong opinions about running and being distracted by listening to music or motivational sessions, which I cover in another chapter. The bottom line is a watch with GPS is nice to have, so if you can afford it, go for it.

So, I've covered the essential running equipment and given you my thoughts on the topic. I've not told you what shoes and clothing and accessories I use. This is because as soon as I put them down into this book, they'll change. Everything changes over a running year. But I also don't want to leave you hanging, so I've compromised and put them up on my companion website for this book. The website name is www.RunToEnjoyLife.com, and you'll find other running resources at the site.

This seems a much better way to provide you the latest on what I'm using and what's available out there. It also means I can give you my thoughts on what has changed and what's new. Who knew today we could walk around with a watch on our wrist that can communicate with satellites thousands of miles in space, know precisely where we are, and give us reasonably accurate information?

So, to recap, an excellent pair of shoes is all you need to enjoy running – but don't go out running in just a pair of shoes! Seriously, everything else beyond the basics, just like life, is trimming and won't make you any happier, just maybe more comfortable. And there's nothing wrong with being more comfortable, but don't get it mixed up with the belief that you can't be happy and content if you don't have the extras. That kind of thinking keeps people imprisoned in unhappiness!

Next up is one of my favorite topics—making your running playful. This is the chapter where your running starts, now that you have your gear, and you're in the mood and prepared to take your first or next running steps.

CHAPTER SIX

The Power of Play

"We don't stop playing because we grow old;
we grow old because we stop playing"
– George Bernard Shaw

Y ou've no doubt heard the term "*all work and no play makes jack a dull boy.*" It's an old proverb about how we become bored and boring to others if our life is only about our work or job or a specific focus. This is true in your running as well, as in all work and no play in your running makes your sessions dull. We want, after all, to look forward to our training and not be so robotic about it we lose sight of why we run.

If all your running comprises the same pre-scheduled workouts done on the same outdoor roads or track, it will eventually feel like work and about as far away from fun as visiting a dentist for a root canal. Even if your body is not bored, then your mind and spirit will become jaded. This is no different from life.

This chapter follows all the ways I've learned to keep my enjoyment of running front and center when out training.

To get us in the right frame of mind, I'll introduce the word *"play"* to encapsulate these ways. I know as a mature adult, the term "*play*" is usually reserved for how you describe the activity for your kids, grandkids, or when you're on vacation or holiday. The word "*play*" as an activity you participate in at work or in your leisure time doesn't quickly spring to mind. As adults, we may use the term fun, but... *play*? It somehow suggests we don't take it seriously. This is far from the truth. I'm suggesting now that play is deadly serious, for some, even lifesaving.

I want you to get into the habit of labeling what follows as "*play*." Because how we label activity is vitally important for how we think about it and the sentiment it conjures up.

A second concept to introduce here is "*creativity*." It's thought that creative people, such as writers, artists, or entertainers, are that way because they've never lost their ability to "*play*." It's what makes them creative and to stay creative. We may even call them geniuses for their ability to create. The rest of us "*lost*" this ability to be creative, and we believe it's gone forever. We had it once— as a child or some fleeting moments as a teenager—now, we point out to others our deficiency in being creative, "*Oh, I'm not creative, but you should see my friend Amy, she's so creative.*"

This just isn't true. You're selling yourself short, believing this. You are born and remain a highly creative individual. Like most, you've just let that side of you lapse, but it's still inside you waiting to be rediscovered and is available to tap back into through play. It's compelling. For more proof on this and a deeper discussion on this topic, check out Steve Chandler's book "*Creator,*" where you can follow him on his search for his creative world.

It's time to get your creativity back and engage it with the play concept to make your running and life more fun.

How do you do this?

Believe it or not, you've lots of options available, and these don't necessarily interfere with any of your goals or training requirements unless you let your head get in the way. I'm going to get you started by sharing what I do, but I recommend adapting and adding to the ones I use.

I'll discuss your options under four topics: *training schedules*, *routes*, *surprises*, and *races*. If you remember, I did warn you about being "*open*" to new approaches and ways of thinking. This is an excellent place to start. In what follows, I'll use the terms "*play*" and "*fun*" interchangeably, depending on the context. I want you to shake up your running routines and add some spice to them.

For many of us, routines are a practical way of dealing with all the decisions we must make to get through one day. Having routines lets our unconscious mind deal with them as habits, so we don't have to think about them. Also, we generally prefer to know what we're doing so we're not startled, surprised, or get our natural balance upset. Depending on your character, you may deal with shake-ups to your routines better than others.

Training Schedule:

Believe it or not, you should schedule fun into your weekly schedule. That's right—schedule it in. If you're a competitive runner, this will make you feel uncomfortable at first, but it's easy to adjust in a way that doesn't impact your performance—at least physically. If you let your head mess with you on it, it can, but that spills over to issues with your belief system, and that is another book.

For me, I schedule fun by choosing to do a long slow run or a short fast run a few times a week. I enjoy both. By the way: I save long fast runs for races; otherwise, somebody will be scraping me off the road.

I make my pace for a long training run slow. If you're with a group, then you should be able to hold a conversation. These are

45

wonderful opportunities to run with a partner who runs slower than you. Your slow running pace may be a stretch for them, but they'll be happy to be pushed. Also, running with others or in a group is a great social opportunity. Heck, I've been in races where it's apparent people are running as a group just like they're out for a Sunday afternoon outing and chatting away and just enjoying being there.

The other option here is a short fast run. I'm not talking about fartlek training but more like... *let me see how fast I can run a mile at the track or on the road.* Here, I'd run slow for two miles for a warm-up—fast mile, but not trying to break a personal record and below a 7-minute pace for me—then easy warm down for 2 miles. Another time, I may decide to do 5 miles tempo pace after a mile warm-up.

It'll be different for you, but you get the picture. If fast is your idea of fun, then schedule it in if you're on a schedule that has you running session after session of slow running to build stamina through aerobic training. Don't get too fixated on mileage if you're just starting. Imprisoning yourself to run the same mileage at the same speed every day for months on end is a sure way to kill any running enthusiasm.

Routes:

I'm a firm believer in changing my scenery whenever I can. Having three or four routes in your repertoire is a necessity to keep boredom at bay. I also look at track as a change of scenery. At one time, going to a track was synonymous with speed work or fast repetitions through interval running. After all, why would you go to a track unless you need to time a specific distance?

But that's false thinking. Going to the track can also mean going slower, especially if you run in the outside lanes and run for time rather than distance. It would be best if you didn't run on the inside lane at a track unless you're doing time trials, as track protocol demands you leave it for others to use for this purpose.

Running in the outside lane also triggers your mind to accept; this isn't an intense training session but a playful one. You can also run clockwise on a track for a change—you'll be surprised how quickly your mind can adapt to going around a track clockwise.

When running on streets and roads, always make loops from your home if you can. Out and back routes can work but making loops means you can run the course reverse, doubling your options for changing things up. Running a familiar route in the reverse direction can feel strange at first, and I guarantee that you'll run slower than expected the first time you do this. But this is just confirmation you are *"playing"* and having *"fun."*

Make sure you've added some routes with hills on them. Hills not only add interest to a course but can provide an excellent anaerobic workout. For more about the terms *"aerobic"* and *"anaerobic,"* see the additional material section toward the end of the book.

Choose your routes carefully and make sure you're never more than 2 – 3 miles to get back home. I have a route that takes me out 3.5 miles, but this pushes my limit if I've got an injury. Injuries happen, and sometimes it's best to stop running and walk home. Having a route that takes you 5 miles to get back home risks further damage and longer recuperation time. I cover this in more detail in another chapter.

Surprises:

How do you surprise yourself on a run? Good question. It doesn't have to be a surprise, like deciding to suddenly sprint hard for 100 yards instead of a fast mile. Sprinting when I'm not ready or prepared is a recipe for disaster for me and likely to result in something *"pulled"* or *"torn."* Neither is suitable for my enjoyment of running or life!

Surprises are more of a considered decision than a split-second one, and I consider how I'm feeling in my running in the first ½ mile or mile of a workout. If my schedule is calling for an easy run of about 5-6 miles, but I feel good, and it seems effortless, and I'm at a 9-minute pace, then I'll keep it going and going. I may not do the entire 5 miles at that pace and ease off the last mile or two, but the point is it becomes a different session than what I started out doing. It can be exhilarating and is a simple way of pushing yourself and being, well… *surprised*.

Like life, we get into a way of keeping everything in its place and tidy, consistent, and… *tedious*. It doesn't take much to spice things up and make running and life enjoyable. You can also do it in small steps.

Races:

Some people only train to race. They wish they could fast-forward to race day. They feel all this time and effort day in and out just to run races and finish a half-marathon, or a full Marathon is… *work*. But they're reminded of all this training they must do! Training becomes a means to an end. They live for the competition, even if the competition is with themselves.

I don't see anything wrong with this, though. It shows the excitement of competition, and I've been there and thought that way in my past. But likely, this isn't you, and you're looking instead to enjoy your workouts. Many of us cringe at the thought of putting ourselves on exhibition and being seen racing, and what if we're seen coming in last? As one runner jokingly put it, coming in at the rear, you get an individual police escort; a personal attendant reserved only for the front leader runner or the last-place finisher. I've rarely been in a race where the spectators don't clap and cheer as loud for those in the rear end as for the winner. Only you care about how you look.

So, entering a race can be enjoyable and does give purpose to your running all those other days of the week. Just like life, looking forward to achieving a race goal is natural. Not having goals makes many of us feel aimless and lost. This may be losing weight or stopping a bad habit or getting a certification in something, going back to school, or visiting another country. The goals are endless, and the fact is, we're engineered to have and achieve goals. It's in our genes and human makeup.

So, pick a running goal and tie it to a race. You don't have to commit to a specific race or date—although, for a half or full marathon, you'll need to have a training schedule in place and start a few months ahead to prepare for being ready. Races and preparing for them then help you keep the fun and the play in your running, and it'll naturally spill over into your life. This is somewhat akin to osmosis, where because you have these positive things happening in one area, it will drift into other areas of your life through your unconscious mind.

We all get into a rut in our life from time to time, which happens in our running as well, so if you feel this way with running, then spice up your workouts to compensate and set a goal for your running if you don't have one to invigorate it.

Of course, the reverse is also true. Don't think all enjoyment is activated from one activity. There will be times when your running is in a rut or not giving you the same pleasure it was before. This may be evidence your life can aid your running by focusing on something outside running to enjoy that you've drifted away from, such as reading, drawing, volunteering, or writing that book you've always wanted to do.

My intent here was to get you thinking differently about enjoying your running through your creative use of play. I've shared my methods and thoughts to start you off. Likely, you can think of other options specific to your personality and preferences. It does require effort and willingness to experiment to keep the spirit of enjoyment going in your running and life. Go to it.

Next up are some mechanics about running outdoors that'll help you enjoy these workouts more while keeping you safe and reducing injuries.

CHAPTER SEVEN

Paying Attention and Avoiding Distractions

"If on any given day you don't cry from rejoicing in the beauty of the world, then you have not lived that day"
— Kamand Kojouri

I've got a picture in my mind of my perfect running day.

It's warm but not hot. It's early morning. The sky is clear, and the sun has just risen. There's a breeze on my beaming face. The natural world is also awakening with birds in song and animals scurrying in the undergrowth. I can even sniff the fragrance of the ponds and the woods on my route. It's a joy to be out running with no other distractions or intrusions of thoughts that take me away from these feelings. It's a perfect day, not just for a run but for my soul.

Your perfect running day may be different from mine. It may be one with a lite cooling rain on your body in a favorite park or around the neighborhood streets of your city. Your sounds and scents are different but still familiar and soothing. Your perfect day may be more about how you feel rather than your environment or the weather.

We share the thought of a perfect day, different though it may be of its constituent parts, it's nonetheless a picture and a feeling we conjure up when asked to describe it. But there are many other days when we run, and they are far from our ideal—overcast and gloomy days with a chilling wind on lonely foreboding roads—runs when our thoughts are troubled, and we're anxious.

Running can help improve all our days if we discover how to pay attention and avoid distractions. In this chapter, I want to discuss two concepts around paying attention and avoiding distractions. One keeps you enjoying your running world, whatever the environment, weather, or mood. The other reduces the risk of injuries.

I'll first focus on enjoyment and why you're outside running and how to ensure you don't lose sight of why you're there. It's more than keeping fit; otherwise, you'd be inside at a gym on a treadmill on bad weather days. Yes, I run for my heart and health, but nature has given us a beautiful outside to explore and appreciate while we do this. It's an ever-changing canvas we begin to paint just for us if we'll just pay attention.

If this all sounds esoteric to you, then this "*paying attention*" is because it's not a part of our emotions we access deliberately often. Recognizing the things that bring us joy during our days full of commitments and rushing from one appointment to another can easily slip from our life as we get more and more distracted by our other routines. We even have a phrase to remind us of its importance, "*stop and smell the roses.*" It takes some effort and focus, but you'll find it quickly becomes easy to pay attention to your world with some practice.

In the summer where I live, even if it's raining, being outside remains pleasant. Warm and keeping you cool running in the rain can be every bit as satisfying as being in the rays of the sun. As I usually run in the morning, especially in the hot summer months, I'm up with the other animals beginning their day to avoid dehydration. I see other folks enjoying the early part of a new day and walkers and occasionally another runner. It helps set my mood for the day. Positive and looking forward to what will unfold.

I'm an early bird. I get up between 5 – 6 AM to start my day. I'm eager to get outside and do my run as early as my schedule allows. I must wait for the sun to rise in the winter, so I usually start my run between 7 am – 8 am. In the summer, I can get out earlier, and this is my preference. When you do, your run for the day will likely be different, but our world can look beautiful anytime in the day if you learn to notice it.

My schedule comprises several slow-distance runs for an hour or longer each week. If you're a beginning runner, it'll take you time to train your body up to this—possibly a year, and this is fine as there's no rush. There's a point in your run, for many around 30/40 minutes, where you'll eventually feel what others call the *"runner's high."* This is where you'll notice the benefits of your running at a different level. It's a euphoric feeling, and you'll be even more attuned to your outside environment. You may even catch yourself smiling and suddenly realize even on a cold, gloomy winter day, all is right with your world.

Your experience, though, will be unique, as will the time the feeling overcomes you. If your temperament is primarily positive, then the change may not be as perceptible in your runs but will happen eventually.

Most of the time, it's to our benefit to avoid distractions when outside running. It avoids competing with appreciating the enjoyment of the outdoors.

Our thoughts can be distracting. Our mind likes to be filled with thoughts as it loathes emptiness. The exact mechanism we don't understand, but you're thinking thoughts even as you read this. I've found focusing on my breathing helps bring me back to the present if I find my thoughts wandering when running. Breathing exercises are often used to combat stress and anxiety, as is running. I'm not suggesting you invoke mindful breathing or Pranayama in the middle of your run, but just deliberately taking in breathes through your nose and exhaling through your mouth, which is the essence of proper breathing anyway. Deliberate breathing requires your attention, so it may help you quiet your mind from racing thoughts to focus more on your outdoors.

Avoiding distractions to me means not running with earbuds. Ask yourself why you need to do this? Is it because you find running boring and want to shut out the world and replace it with something else? Yes, you can walk and chew gum at the same time. But should you? But then why ruin a run by taking yourself to another world? Having some background music can be soothing and help concentrate on other things, but this is surely reserved for a safer environment, such as sitting down at home or riding a bus or the subway.

Even worse for me is listening to podcasts or motivation sessions when out running. Really? This indeed requires you to "*listen*" and think and… be distracted. This is like texting and driving, and we all know where that leads. If you must avoid being in your running, you're just doing it for fitness, and while this is okay, be aware of what you're missing.

So, now I want to move onto the concept of paying attention and avoiding distractions to reduce the risk of injuries.

I choose my routes carefully to avoid highways and traffic as much as possible. Avoiding direct car fumes isn't only good for my body but avoids situations where drivers, particularly in the early morning hours, may not be expecting a runner on the road. While it's not always possible to avoid a busy street, I do my best to minimize how long I stay on them.

Roads can be a dangerous place to run. If there's a path available, then this is the first choice. But in rural areas in America, I've found they're just not available. Sidewalks stop quickly after getting outside residential communities, and you're forced to run in the drains and gutter domain. For the most part, this is fine, but there is danger lurking in these areas with debris and unevenness that can trick you into thinking all is well when in fact, your next step can end up causing a foot or ankle injury.

Paying attention means looking ahead down the immediate road, so you're aware of what will be under your next step. It can just take a twig or stone to displace your foot and make for an awkward landing. It seems each next step needs to be carefully planned to avoid injury. But it's not as complicated as it sounds—your subconscious takes care of most of this for you if you focus on the road.

I've had my missteps.

One wrong step on the road in winter decades ago as a youth meant two months of no running and a missed chance to represent my county for cross country running in the UK. The same sort of misstep in America in the fall months, decades later, kept me out of running for the same amount of time. The first injury was caused during night running, something I never do now. Indeed, I couldn't see the hazard and got too close to the curb when doing interval speed work on the road. Other injuries were under different circumstances—one was caused by tiredness, and another was running through trails in the woods with uneven ground.

Running in New England during the winter months—and we've got a long winter here—increases the risk of accidents. Slippery conditions and any days when the temperature dips below or hovers around freezing tempts spills and injuries to the head, arms, and shoulders. I avoid running with snow underneath my feet. Again, it comes down to not being able to see what is under my next step. After a storm, I'll wait a few days before going outside, and then only if the snow has been cleared and the road has had time to dry out. Running when the thermometer hovers around freezing, though, means ice underneath lurks at each step.

My routes are full of undulating terrain, which I enjoy as it provides some tests for me and adds interest to my runs, but I've found hills have surprises for us as well. Running downhill demands you to be careful even in fair weather but in poor and icy conditions, even more so. As most runners do, running downhill is more jarring on my bones and joints than running uphill. You're more likely to get injured running downhill than up. As they say in racing circles, attack uphill but coast downhills.

Back to my avoidance of running wearing earphones, they interfere with my enjoyment and lessen my awareness of my surroundings and approaching vehicles. Even in ideal conditions, drivers have all sorts of things to distract them. They don't necessarily expect to see a runner sharing their road with them. If your earbuds are muffling the sound of their approaching engine, then your next step, deviating from where you were a few steps before, means a driver can be surprised and not have time to avoid you. Whatever the scenario you paint, it isn't a pleasant outcome for you.

We learn early in running on roads that you should always try and face oncoming traffic. The Road Runners Club of America recommends you run against traffic. This also allows you to see car or motorcycle headlights in poor lighting conditions. As far as I know, no laws govern this, but it makes sense to me to, whenever possible, follow this guidance. Some states provide codes about walking and running and require sidewalks to be used if available and only cross at intersections or marked crosswalks. Where there is a code in your state or town or whatever country you live in, then know the rules of the road for running on them.

Occasionally, running on the side of the road recommended is challenging. It can have more undergrowth and debris than the other side, which may be clearer and safer to run on. I've also found sharp bends where you can't see vehicles coming around. They can't see you either; they have produced a few "*close shaves*" for me. I adjust by slowing down and listening for an approaching vehicle. If forced to run with the flow of traffic, be more vigilant and make sure to minimalize these times and cross over to face the traffic at your first safe opportunity.

It may seem obvious, but it does help to wear reflective clothing in poor light conditions. I'm not talking about just when going out at night or running at dusk and dawn but during the day in foul weather. Good quality running shoes will have reflective stripes, as will clothing, and this adds a layer of protection to be seen by drivers.

Bad weather days, including stormy days, can also hide dangers under puddles. I know my routes well and where the larger puddles accumulate and avoid roads where small ponds suddenly appear at the slightest downpour near drains or in poor drainage areas. Not only do drivers need to swerve, but you may also need to perform a similar maneuver, so paying attention is required. Also, I'm not particularly eager to run through deep puddles. I'd instead stop and run around them if all is clear than have my socks and feet wet for the next 30 or 60 minutes of running, especially in cold weather. Losing heat while running in any of my body extremities makes me miserable and lessens the run's enjoyment.

Pay attention in residential areas for cars reversing out of driveways. This is a particular hazard for me as my running is primarily early morning when people leave for work or school.

Again, drivers aren't expecting an approaching runner as they reverse out into the street. Usually, I can see and hear the engine and have time to slow down and avoid them, but I've had several near misses on quiet neighborhood roads.

So, to recap, get out and enjoy your running by listening to the world outside. Enjoy the sights and sounds and be part of the present in your environment. Pay attention and avoid distractions to enjoy your runs and to keep safe. Watch out for vehicles on the road and don't pick an argument with them; avoid them and run defensively.

My next topic will show you how running can help lift your spirits and prepare you for a second crack at having one of the best days of your life.

CHAPTER EIGHT

Rainy Mornings and Sunny Afternoons

"The greater part of our happiness or misery depends upon our dispositions, and not upon our circumstances."
– Martha Washington

I grew up in a temperate climate where there seemed more rainy days than sunny ones, but running on tracks, fields, and roads in any type of weather never seemed to impact my pleasure for it. The biting, bone-chilling winds of a wet English winter can compete with any day I've run in a bitter, dry, cold New England.

But that's about the actual weather, and that's just one part of the story in this chapter. Sprinkled in with the impact of actual weather conditions is how we feel on any given day. What's on our mind and in our thoughts. Metaphorically, we often attach how we feel to weather conditions. We experience "*rainy days*" in our lives even when the sun is shining outside. An event or circumstances can cause us to lose morale, or darkness can overtake our thoughts, and we become anxious and even in despair. The opposite is also true. Our spirits can be "*sunny*" despite a raging storm outside, and it seems nothing can dampen our spirits.

We can describe our running days then as rainy and sunny for the weather and our moods. The actual weather we can't do much about. It is what it is. Our moods, though, we can influence, and running can help us to do this.

I don't run outdoors in weather that's unsafe for me. Apart from the obvious scenarios such as snow and lightning storms to stay indoors, I'll not run outside if road conditions or visibility are poor or slippery. As mentioned in a previous chapter, I've got a few routes that become hazardous during heavy or prolonged rain, so I avoid those altogether or sections of them.

While I may feel confident about navigating my routes during adverse conditions, I remain skeptical drivers will be on the lookout for me. Distractions and visibility issues for them increase my risk with their inability to navigate these conditions. So, knowing when to stay off the roads for your survival comes down to good choices. I'm not a fanatic when it comes to running, and I don't adopt a *"must-run"* mentality every day my schedule says, or I feel I've let myself down and allow a negative mood to overtake me. I prefer to reframe the situation and tell myself I'm saving *"me"* for another day. I'm not one of those who can, or need to, exclaim, *"I've not missed a day of running in 10 years."*

Rainy mornings can set the tone for a day. I don't mind running in the rain. In fact, in the hot summer months, it can be a relief, and anyway, after the first mile of a run, you're sweating enough that keeping dry is a lost cause. Rain during a long training session is welcome to me. Poor weather days don't dampen my spirits. The world and your environment rejoice in the rain as it provides life to animals and plants you share your running routes with.

Accepting rainy starts to the day and its benefits then positions you to enjoy your run in those conditions. I may change my schedule based on the weather. If the rain is hard, choosing a long run rather than a fast or interval session may make sense to you unless you've access to a track. Increased vigilance on a wet road may compete for your attention over monitoring your speed and keeping track of repeats. It's easy to lose count of repetitions even when not distracted—is this number 5 of 10, or am I on number 6? It happens.

This change in your type of run based on conditions comes back to being flexible again. The goal is to get to the end of the session feeling good and not injured.

There are days when the weather is foul or miserable, winter days come to mind, and it's hard to think positive and enjoy them compared to other runs. You just want to get through it and on to the rest of your day.

So, weather conditions are one element, but your attitude and thoughts are quite another. You may have something on your mind. Yesterday may not have been the best day of your life. It lingers with you overnight and into the morning. You need time to work things through or put them to rest. Your thoughts and feelings can create the atmosphere of a gloomy rainy morning.

Whatever the reasons hidden within my training routine are an opportunity to start or split the day into two. Don't think halves but sections that aren't measured to any length of time.

Letting your training run take over your mood to get lost in your session and take you out of your current *"rainy"* mood can take some work. Our thoughts get in the way all the time. They linger and overtake our run if we let them and cloud our enjoyment. If you're the type of person who will allow these thoughts to eat you up and keep reminding yourself of just how bad the previous day was or is being today, then try reframing.

Reframing is a way of changing negative intrusive thoughts with happy ones. Most of us have a lot of positive good stuff happening in our lives, but it's easy to allow a negative experience to magnify and take over our entire world. We can also linger in a thought process that assumes we know the outcome, and we paint it black, but it's unlikely it'll ever be as bad as we think. We play a movie in our head or a discussion with an antagonist over and over thinking we'll get a different ending but don't. We take things personally when we shouldn't, as other people have bad days and what they said, or did, had nothing to do with you. Reframing as we run when negative thoughts overtake us can be achieved by simply choosing different thoughts to focus on.

I come back to breathing again to help to refocus my thoughts. Deliberately focusing on proper breathing when running— breathe through the nose and out the mouth—works to expel whatever thoughts dictate a sour mood quickly. I can't do one while thinking about the other.

Accept you'll not be able to enjoy every run you have to the same degree. After all, if every day were sunny, then you'd not have any sunny days to look forward to. If every day was perfect, then perfect becomes normal. Learn to deal with the imperfect days and use your running to cope with them.

During my professional working life, I frequently had the opportunity to run at lunchtime. For those of you who work at home, this may work for you as well. It's not a bad time to run. It does mean finding a way of taking in food after your session and sometimes perspiring long after your shower, but for some, this is preferable to trying to fit it in before or after work.

I looked at being able to run at lunchtime as splitting my day into two halves. A positive and good morning could, after my run, continue or be even better. A morning that wasn't so great for me could be turned around by resetting my attitude for the afternoon. I could brush aside effectively my *"rainy morning"* with my run and get into a *"sunny afternoon,"* metaphorically speaking. This split of the day works well for a lunchtime run. But not everybody runs at lunchtime or can.

So, what then?

I prefer to run in the morning as early as possible, depending on my schedule for the day. Like most, I don't always have the luxury of scheduling my day around my run. I've also had times in my life when running after my workday finished was the only way I'd get my session in. This I found the most difficult, as it interrupted family time and my eating habits. Eating a family dinner in the evening after my run and shower when my appetite was low was not ideal for my body or nutrition. It also didn't help to split my day in two the way other scenarios did, such as morning or lunchtime sessions.

But for you, running after work may be ideal, especially if your main meal is at lunchtime and you don't have commitments in the evening—different strokes for different folks and phases of your life.

The whole point here is to use your running session to push your refresh button for the day.

Using your running session to change your mood is also based on science. When you run, it reduces your body's stress hormones such as adrenaline and cortisol and stimulates the production of endorphins which are chemicals that are natural mood elevators. So, running, along with other aerobic exercise activities, can scientifically help you reset your day.

In full disclosure, hard training sessions or long runs can cause an increase in your cortisol level, which is to be avoided regularly. However, athletes' current thinking is used sparingly; then, it can make you stronger and improve performance. Additionally, as your body strength increases and your fitness level rises, you can condition your body to accommodate more long runs.

I tend to do one long run once a week. My long run is about 13 – 15 miles, and I always rest the next day, and my hard run tends to be two sessions per week of tempo and fartlek sessions at around a fast or race pace. If your focus is about enjoying your running and not being competitive, then there's little evidence to suggest infrequently running hard will increase your cortisol level. But you should do your research, come to your conclusions, and adjust your schedule for your capabilities and goals.

Again, I'm all about the enjoyment of my running, and I don't get hung-up about adjusting on the fly based on how I feel and what my body is telling me on the day. Alternatively, there's nothing wrong with pushing yourself on some of your runs to improve and test your running progress. I've found when I push, I surprise myself and am usually capable of achieving something I didn't expect, especially in races and sometimes in workouts.

When I lived in more urban areas, then I sought out parks to run it. My lunchtime runs when working in Boston were routed along the Charles River. Usually, you can improvise, and while you may not be able to get to the silence you prefer, you can generally find routes in urban areas where it's safe and protected. You can enjoy being outdoors without the constant city and traffic noises.

There are other ways of hitting your reset button for the day with your running.

Learning to love the outdoors isn't just about nature and wildlife but also about discovery and being observant. If you learn to become aware of your environment, you'll be surprised at what you missed right in front of you before. A slight detour on a road you've never taken before can lead you to an undiscovered trail or a scenic and tranquil street. Finding treasures you never knew existed can add enjoyment by taking you away from your well-trodden path to visit a new and different scenic backdrop.

I tend to reserve this exploration for my long run day, which is usually Sunday. This provides me the opportunity to absorb these adventures from a time perspective. On weekdays, I typically have other commitments which don't offer me the time of experimentation. But on my long-run days, I can afford to have a few dead ends without impacting the rest of my day.

I've discussed how to utilize your session to split up your day and get the benefits of changing moods and attitudes so your day becomes more enjoyable even in those *"rainy day morning"* scenarios so you can get to more *"sunny afternoons."* It's just another way of looking at the impact your running can have on your life.

Next up, I share what has worked for me in reducing and recovering from injuries and provide some alternative thoughts about myths and advice out there, which might leave you confused and frustrated.

CHAPTER NINE

Reducing and Recovering from Injuries

"Almost all accidents and injuries happen when
an individual is not being present and not
paying attention to what they are doing."
– Tobe Hanson

The best type of injury is the one that doesn't happen. I'd rather prevent injuries than suffer through them with all the physical pain and mental anguish that comes with the misery ride.

I've been fortunate enough not to have many injuries in my running life, and I fully intend for that to continue as I age further. And when I talk about injuries, I mean those that force you out of running for a month or longer, rather than muscle stiffness or aches that disappear after skipping workouts for a day or two.

I can vividly recall four significant injuries that have kept me from pounding the pavement for long spells. Compared to the number of years I've been running, this is a small number. The most major of these was a knee injury sustained in a training run that caused a rehabilitation period of the best part of a year. This one stopped me from running and required a visit to a sports clinic for diagnosis and resolution. I know exactly how it happened and, to a certain extent, why.

I had participated in a team relay in New Hampshire. It was called "*Reach the Beach.*" It's a relay of different distances over 24 hours. Each runner in my team had two legs of different lengths, starting in the White Mountains and running to Hampton Beach, a town close to the Massachusetts border.

I had my first relay leg early on, about 4/5 miles, and then another overnight of slightly longer distance. I felt fine after my relay legs were completed. I'd some soreness in my leg muscles by the end of my second relay leg, which was overnight, but that was to be expected. I learned a few days later that the relay had exposed a weakness in my knees that had been building up for a while. Knees are common weak points for runners. My lurking injury suddenly surfaced during my first workout a few days after the relay race. I went out intending a leisurely pace to "*run the soreness*" out of my legs.

However, my right knee completely gave out just a few minutes into my run but luckily less than a mile from home. No warning, just a complete collapse of my right leg. I knew instantly it was severe. I ended up in a heap in the middle of a quiet road, just staring at the knee, fearing to put any weight on it. It's one of those injuries that, when it happens, your thoughts automatically rush to the worst-case scenario. Is this the injury that needs an operation? Will I ever be able to run again? Will this injury confine me to another activity I won't enjoy as much?

Eventually, I realized I needed to get home. I could hardly hobble, let alone walk. Though less than ½ mile from home, it seemed to take ages to nurse myself back home, shuffling step by step, fearful of the damage I could be doing to the knee by putting any weight on it. No sports cart from Gillette Stadium arrived to take me into a locker room for immediate expert attention. Just my somber thoughts as company on my return trip home. A season-ending injury for sure.

This injury kept me out of running for many months. I had a specialist at a sports clinic provide a prognosis, and both knees had the patella (kneecap) slightly out of alignment. Physiotherapy, but lucky for me, no surgery was prescribed. The following months were spent performing a rote set of exercises to reset the patella on both legs to their normal positions. Eventually, I was able to cycle as part of my recovery and got back to full running capabilities within a year. It was a long despondent year before I could make another entry in my running logbook.

My other injuries were ankle twists and sprain caused when tired, under poor conditions, or on rugged trails and not paying attention. Now you understand why I repeatedly advocate for you to pay attention when running. Today, my first way of reducing injury recognizes the signs when I'm at risk and play safety first. Before any workout, I stretch.

I admit I don't particularly enjoy stretching. I'd much prefer to step outside and close the front door and start my run immediately. But I know I've weak spots in my running frame, and an ounce of prevention can save me months of recovery by preparing for my run. Stretching before and after my workout takes a few minutes and can help pinpoint issues. There's a body of research that concludes stretching doesn't prevent injuries. But I'm not a statistic and continue to stretch. I watch Olympic and champion athletes stretch and folks who punish their bodies much more than I go through their stretching ritual. I figure they know more than me. So, even if just for my mental preparation, I stretch before every run.

But stretching isn't my only preparation before a workout. I also perform a self-check. This covers a physical and mental check-in with "*me*." How do I feel? Any soreness or tightness? Do I feel tired? Am I alert and focused, or am I distracted and less than attentive? How do I feel when I do my stretching or warm-up jog before a race? Can I still feel yesterday's run? I know I can nearly always feel some stiffness from the previous day until I run it out of my legs, but there's a difference between stiffness and a constant leg ache.

It doesn't stop in my warm-up period either. When I'm out running, I'm constantly performing the same ongoing checks. If my leg tiredness hasn't left me within the first mile, then there's usually a reason, and a shorter run than scheduled that day would be better for me. If I'm due to perform interval/fartlek speed work, then there may be a need to reconsider. This isn't as complicated as it sounds. Most of it is evident at the start of your workout. The problematic aspect is deliberate listening to what your body is telling you. Running in a group or with a partner who has gotten out of bed early to make a workout date with you puts pressure on you to do the run regardless. But the workout can be different based on how you feel.

All of us feel twinges when running. These are muscle spasms that can happen at any time as our body adjusts to conditions or what we're asking it to do. They don't usually last more than a few steps. If they do, they demand our attention, especially in races, when we're pushing ourselves harder than usual for a sustained period. Easing off the pace can help with twinges or even stopping for a few minutes if persisting. While twinges can turn into something more serious, this is rare. Like side stitches, you can usually run through them.

When running, avoiding injury can take several forms. Listening to your body and what it's telling you and acting on it. By the end of your first mile, you can usually tell how things are going and whether to continue or not. I call it the "*is today a good day for a good run?'* check. Is my body up to the demands? What are the conditions like? Considering how I feel and my environment, then should I continue or go home?

I'm nowadays realistic with myself. I can afford to be as I don't have anybody or any reason pushing me. It's all up to me. It's my body at risk, not some other person's. When it comes to running, I'm not *"lazy"* or *"soft."* I consider myself hardy, but I'm experienced and have just been there and done it to my body for all the wrong reasons and paid the price. And it's not worth it. Not running on a scheduled day is still a disappointment to me. But it comes back to we're in this to enjoy running and life. Whether I run 30 or 60 miles this week isn't going to make a physical difference to my fitness or health.

On those rare days of needing to skip a session, I can console myself with a long walk if the thought of doing nothing prays on my conscience. Providing we're just talking about tiredness and not a painful injury, then a long walk outdoors is the next best thing to a run, and it's good for the soul as well. Walking the same day as a run can help me avoid leg soreness or tiredness the next day.

Alertness plays a vital role in keeping injury-free. Paying attention when running or anticipating situations is, of course, key when out on the roads. Avoid situations that place you at risk. If you're distracted, either due to work or personal reasons causing your mind to wander instead of focusing on your next step, then bring yourself back to the present when you realize this. If it keeps happening, then accept you're not alert to dangers that day and get yourself home.

Look out for distracted drivers and run defensively. Most drivers will see you if you're running against their flow as it gives them longer to avoid you if you're not on the sidewalk. Distracted drivers, however, usually aren't giving you a wide berth by changing their course. This is another reason for running against their flow. You can see if they've recognized you're there by giving you a wider berth of the road. If they haven't seen you or are being squeezed by another car coming on the other side of the road, most will slow down to help both them and you pass without contact. If it's obvious they haven't seen you, then that's the time to take evasive action and stop running and step aside.

We can all get distracted, and it doesn't matter who's in the right or wrong; the point at that moment is to preserve yourself. You can curse the driver later when you're still in one piece.

Avoid puddles like the plague when out running. You don't know what lurks submerged. A puddle, even small ones, can hide a pothole or a stick or stone waiting to twist your ankle or jar a knee.

I run a lot on rural roads with residential homes and long driveways. Cars reversing out of their driveways into the street are prime accident maneuvers for runners. Drivers are not expecting a runner to be in their path. They're usually not even looking in my direction, being concerned about colliding with another car rather than a runner. Again, this is all defensive running when on the road.

So, what happens when you do get injured? With the best will in the world, you'll at some point suffer an injury. If you're out running and get injured or have an accident, then your first concern is getting home. Assuming it's not a life-threatening situation, you should seek help if you can't walk back home. Many runners take their phone out with them, and a quick call to family or friends for a ride prevents more damage.

I wear an ID bracelet with an emergency contact number on it. This isn't an expensive device but can help get you aid if you become incapacitated, especially when out on a long solo run or in a race where you can become disorientated or exhausted and need attention from others. Many marathon races offer this as a service when you sign-up.

Many times, for muscle and joint injuries, you'll be able to nurse yourself home if it's a walk of just one or two miles back. If there's no one to help you get home and you're forced to walk and potentially do more damage to your injury, then it'll likely mean a more extended recovery period. The main goal is to get home as quickly and safely as you can so you can start recovery.

Frustrating though it is, know you can't, and shouldn't, rush recovery from any injury. If it's a recurring injury, then you'll know what to do. In other instances, don't hesitate to seek out a doctor's exam and advice or a specialist at a sports clinic.

As in my case, I could've avoided a long recuperation period by attending to the warning signs in my knees earlier and knowing I wasn't prepared enough to perform two relay stints in one day. I ended up in rehabilitation for many months doing exercises each day on mats. And when I started running again, I'd a regimen for months of mostly walking and short duration running. My physiotherapy exercises with foam rollers only got me so far on the road back to running.

In the end, I had to give my body time to heal itself and, during this period, find alternative exercise options to avoid losing all the progress I'd made on my fitness. I joined a gym where I could use equipment to strengthen my legs on a stationary cycle. You may decide a rowing machine or swimming are better alternatives for you on your road back to full recovery.

Personally, using gym equipment or alternative sports doesn't float my boat. During these injury recovering periods, I can't wait to get back to running and the liberation of being outdoors on my favorite routes.

Lest you feel I'm against all non-running gym work, then there's one area where you'll benefit from weights and resistance equipment. As you get older, you naturally lose muscle mass, particularly in your upper body. Doing weight or resistance band exercises can help improve muscle gain and reduce muscle loss and deterioration. But I do this in addition to my running and not instead of any of my sessions.

If you want to explore more options in this area, check out my website at www.RunToEnjoyLife.com, where you can see my evaluations and what products I currently use.

I want to cover one more topic here, as it's common to many runners and athletes who perform an intensive exercise and can easily overextend themselves without realizing it. Your body can develop internal injuries, particularly related to blood in the urine. If you experience this, then don't panic but get it checked out immediately. It can be caused by insufficient recovery time between workouts, or, as I said, overextending yourself, or dehydration issues. This was particularly a problem for me in the hot summer months when training for my first marathon. This is yet another reason for being gentle on your body and not doing too much too soon, be it the number of miles per week or back-to-back intense workouts.

So, we've covered how I keep myself relatively injury and pain-free and my suggestions on recovery. I'm not a sports doctor or a physician. I use my own experience and common sense and seek professional advice and recommendations when dealing with a running-related injury. But at the end of the day, my advice is to adopt routines and protocols based on prevention.

The following section discusses avoiding *"burnout"* in your running. Burnout can manifest itself in many ways and results in injury, staleness, and a lack of enjoyment. So, before you meet this unfriendly antagonist who takes the edge off your running and can drive you to hang up your shoes for good, get my lowdown on how to avoid and recover from it.

CHAPTER TEN

Avoiding "Burnout" But Keeping the Edge

*"Burnout is not the result of doing too much; it is
the result of not getting enough rest."*
– John Patrick Hickey

Burnout happens when we put our body under stress for an extended period with no release. It's a term often related to work and employment. Most of us can conjure up the name of a colleague or friend, or two who reached a state of physical or emotional exhaustion. Somebody who ignored the warning signs and ended up on the human equivalent of the auto junkyard. Broken. But we only get one body, one vehicle to get through life. No trade-in for a fresh model is available.

High-profile and stressful jobs are typical these days. We trade hours for money and neglect recreation, relationships, and taking care of ourselves. Eventually, the body and the soul pay the price. Making money and having a fabulous lifestyle tied to a job or career can quickly become like a prison—the wrong kind of treadmill.

When it comes to exercise and fitness, then we can quickly slip into the equivalent of burnout on our body and mind. We can easily overdo it as we push ourselves beyond our capabilities in an attempt to be the best athlete we can be, at the expense of everything else. Running becomes our obsession and life. We live to run. We put up with the hassles at work and the demands of relationships so we can get to our running and the place where we're the happiest. But in the process, we lose our balance of life, and eventually, if we don't recognize what's happening, our enjoyment of running—the reason we started this journey in the first place.

It's not like one day we're content with running and the next in despair over it. Instead, the burnout is insidious. Training becomes more like work and no play. Your body always feels tired. You're in a rut and feeling stale. You don't feel right. You find reasons to skip a session or two. You go on vacation or a trip and can't be bothered to pack your running gear with you. You begin to second guess if running for you has run its course and contemplate moving onto your next challenge.

But you're made of sterner stuff. You're not like the folks in the 1970s and 80s who eventually left running looking for the next fad in exercise. Running wasn't a way of life for them. They moved on when the next shiny object appeared. But you're different. You're happy to be outside in a group or with your own company and thoughts, just running and doing your therapy.

But burnout can be real. It happened to me, and worse, I didn't understand what was happening and had nobody to explain what was going on and how to keep the running flame burning inside me. But you do, and so what follows, hopefully, is some help.

As we're more than our job, then we're more than an athlete. Those who can recognize this along the journey can choose a better path to become the best-balanced person they want to be in their life for themselves and those they care about. I believe runners come in all shapes and sizes and temperaments. I don't subscribe to the convenient categorization that all distance runners are scrawny and frail-looking and shun the social life preferring a solitary path. This is just not true. The runners I've known aim for a balanced life and don't fit into one mold.

So, what causes burnout in running?

There are a few obvious reasons I've experienced and seen. Demanding schedules with insufficient recovery or breaks. The monotony of doing the same thing day in and day out 6/7 days a week without results or improvement. No goals or races to act as a path to continue with excitement. Not sharing our running and hopes and dreams with others, and instead detached and alone.

As I mentioned, I experienced burnout when I was younger. I pushed myself to run 100 miles a week when young. There wasn't time for much else in my life except work and running. After all, do the math yourself, averaging over 14 miles per day, seven days a week, and a 9-hour workday with a commute doesn't leave room for much else.

Why did I do this?

It was the days of the 100 miles a week training schedules. The elite were doing it, and I wanted to associate with that band of runners. So, I assumed to be a legitimate card-carrying member of that club; I needed to do what they were doing. But my body wasn't conditioned and ready, and I didn't know how to manage the mental aspect that came with it. Indeed, I'd worked up to 60/70 miles a week over a few years, but taking my mileage up a few notches to 100 miles a week made me constantly tired. I also trained hard most days and had few easy workouts. Many times, my training runs were faster than my races.

I'd try and figure out what I was doing wrong for long periods, constantly tired, not getting the results I wanted. Sound familiar? Your body can only take that kind of punishment for so long before fighting back. As I didn't see the fruits of my labor for long periods, I began to make other life changes, and my love of running begun to wane. I found reasons to skip sessions, and over time I began to find my enjoyment in other activities.

I had reached "*burnout*" with my running. I left it all in my training sessions and had nothing left for races or life. Life became difficult because I identified as a runner, but I drifted away from this identity.

I had a break from running, but this proved to be a blessing in disguise for me. Getting over the physical burnout was the easiest part for me. The physical body heals quickly. But the mental train wreck took longer to untangle and clear. Putting the wheels back on the track takes longer.

The time between inactivity and restart healed the burnout as a different perspective came into view. A mindset that rebels against feeling life is passing you by, or somebody else controls your life. I eventually returned to my running because I had to. It fulfilled a need in my life.

I didn't return because I was missing the thrill of the race or competition with others. I was missing the void in my life distance running filled. I believe there are interests in our life that speak outside what we do for work and our role as a spouse, parent, sibling, or friend. To have discovered these interests and to be able to pursue them is a gift at whatever stage in our life they appear or reappear in my case.

So, I came back to my running with a different attitude. But more than just an attitude; also an approach to guard against any burnout recurrence. This approach was all about being gentle with the physical and mental aspects of my running. Sharing and balancing my running with my life instead of the single-minded attitude of my youth's ultra-competitive days.

It can take time to work things out in your head on what's important and how to implement it. It's easy to lose track and get wrapped up in an activity, especially if you expect the best from yourself every time. I've known runners who approach every training session hard. They don't know how to have an easy session and, more perplexing to them, why you'd want to. But I realized this was not me. If it ever was, it was no longer.

If I train for a marathon or shorter distance races, I'll do the miles to gain the confidence that I've got the stamina to complete it. I'll push myself in training to experience a race pace for a while but not run the race. I approach each workout now to enjoy it, be it to take it easy or run swiftly. Each outcome can be pleasing if I remember I'm not a machine and set my expectations on this premise and the day.

But what of this *"edge"* I alluded to earlier?

The edge guards against burnout. It takes the causes and offers prevention. It sprinkles easy runs or rest days with demanding days on your schedule. It mixes in play during workouts to keep it interesting. It changes things up on location, routes, and surfaces to combat monotony. It encourages having goals and entering races to add excitement and measure progress. Finally, it embraces discussing your running with those you care about— family, friends, other runners, work colleagues. Even though distance running is an individual sport, we can, and should, share the importance of it with others.

Keeping the edge to me is about keeping your running interesting in your life in all its facets. It's not about running controlling your life, but the opposite. It's us that provides the meaning of running in our life. For me, this is to keep it in its sacred place and focus on doing what I can to keep the anticipation of going out for my next run eager. Each run of each day is an opportunity to prepare for the next run. A chance to look back after the workout is over and be able to smile for the satisfaction it provides.

It doesn't mean there aren't days when it would be easier to skip and do something else… and when I need to, I do. The body and the soul need to be listened to in the court of fair hearing before putting on your shoes. Your resolve and overcoming inertia are cards to play to get out and run, but protection and prevention are different looking, though an equally important and valid hand to play.

People worry about skipping a day. Runners boast they've never missed a day of training in the last decade. It's worn like a red badge of courage. What are we saying here? Is this for our benefit or just bragging rights? Does our body or soul care? Is it that important in who we are or what we have become to somehow measure our life by our ability to do something day in and day out and feel that is it?

I haven't enjoyed every run I've ever done in my life. Some of my races have been downright miserable. But these runs today are few and far between. I give myself permission to not have great runs every day and not let it deter me from putting on my shoes the following day.

Today I feel no qualms about skipping a training session as life demands take over or other commitments conflict with my schedule. I don't let a schedule dictate my life. It's only a map to a destination, and I can take detours to get there. Nobody gets hurt because I don't run. I permit myself to play hooky to keep the enjoyment alive. I've trusted in myself; it's just for the day, and tomorrow I'll participate in my scheduled run because I'll miss it otherwise.

Maybe this isn't you. Perhaps you don't trust yourself, and skipping a day becomes two then three, and before you wake up to it, the whole week has disappeared, and you haven't missed it?

So, maybe there's something else going on in your life needing attention? You may even think, *"well, maybe I don't enjoy running as much as I thought I did? It's become a burden, yet another tug on my time."*

To me, superficially, it suggests you need to slack off for a while to avoid *"burnout."* To keep doing the same thing hoping one day you'll enjoy it, is a recipe for *"burnout."* There's no harm in taking some of the self-imposed stress out of your running and life. Give yourself permission to relax and recuperate if needed. Just be honest and authentic with yourself on the reasons why running takes those occasional back-seat days.

Keeping the edge can be deciding to do a particular race, so you need to implement a training schedule in preparation for it. It could be about doing some cross-training and adding other forms of exercise to your regime. This could be muscle-building routines we've discussed already in other chapters, such as swimming or rowing on a machine, resistance training, or going out for bike rides. Other exercise forms can be creative periods for us all.

I often walk on my rest days which could be unscheduled or not. Walking with somebody else can be beneficial. Walking to think things through is a common experience for me. Sometimes I do it on my own, and other times with a family member or whoever will listen to me.

I execute my schedule to keep my edge by changing things up, sometimes planned or just on the fly, and based on how I feel. After all, I'm not doing this for anybody else but me. Running is purely selfish.

I had a long spell when returning from my knee injury of countless training sessions of a modified interval schedule that involved walking and running. I would walk for 2 minutes and then run as hard as I could for one minute. While I'm no speed merchant and find running fast hard, I figured I could push myself on speed for one minute. Then walk for two. I'd work myself up to be able to do about 5 or 6 repeats of this in a session. Far from being easy, it's intense, but you know you can get through as it's manageable bites. You're not setting out on a training run for 30 minutes or an hour of aerobic or anaerobic reps—just 60 seconds of a speed run. Additionally, if you keep a brisk pace while walking, you can do an intensive session in just 20 minutes. I still engage this twist on a workout as needed.

But the point is, you have the freedom to hit refresh on your running anytime you want if you feel you're becoming stale— anything to avoid burnout. But you are keeping the edge.

So, we come to the final point in this section. Your running is going great. You've found enjoyment in it, but it doesn't seem to be helping with your enjoyment of life. It's not spilling over. It's become a sanctuary rather than enabling you to enjoy your life more.

What is this? What's going on?

Yes, it happens. My promise isn't that running cures all ills. It can undoubtedly be a therapeutic aid. My premise is that having enjoyment in your life, such as running, can add to your happiness. It's not in place of your life. It can become an enabler to appreciating life generally. How you tackle and balance your running provides lessons to take into other areas of your life.

But it's valid if there are situations in your life that demand your attention and focus, and running is primarily there for you as a sanctuary while you work through those circumstances. Only you can make those decisions of what and how to address them. My whole point is to let running play a part in your life that makes sense for you and supports you.

It's, after all, only running. Vital as it is to me in my enjoyment, I've never in my later years let it be something to do instead of attending to life situations needing my focus and attention, particularly when it comes to family and my well-being.

So, we've talked about different forms of *"burnout"* and how to avoid it or recognize it and back off—how to give yourself permission to cope and change to stop becoming bored. We've also acknowledged there's value in making sure your routines don't end up making you feel stale but help you keep the edge in your running to make it exciting and spill over into your life.

You'll find your way to reach the same spot I've reached. Your path, though, may necessarily be different than mine.

Next up, we'll talk about nutrition, how it plays into your enjoyment, and how it can help with injuries and keep your body in tip-top shape. Nutrition is a complicated topic, so I'll keep it simple and give you some food for thought.

CHAPTER ELEVEN

Fuel for Your Running Body

"Thou shouldst eat to live; not live to eat."
- Socrates

I t seems to me the use of common sense is vastly overlooked when it comes to what we put in our body and expect it to do.

We quickly learn about gravity as a kid. Lose your balance on a bike, and you crash to the ground. Putting your hand into the lion cage is not good for your hand. Boiling water burns the skin. As an adult, if we never change the oil in our car, one day, it will seize. None of this is that complicated. Think simple cause and effect.

But when it comes to food—what supplies the energy not only to keep us alive but also dictates the quality of life and health— all common sense goes out the window. We essentially rely on the food industry to tell us what's good for us. This is akin to letting the fox guard the henhouse.

Healthy food choices are a road less traveled for many, and I've certainly taken a few detours during my life to get to where I am today. Let me come clean on a few things at the start. I grew up a meat and potatoes kid. I shuffled my vegetables around on the plate the same as many other kids of my era. Fruit was for scrumping (*kid's pastime for "stealing fruit" from neighbors' trees*), but you never ate the spoils of your play. I love candy and cake— even as an adult.

I'm not a qualified nutritionist or a medical doctor, but neither of these professionals offers much help to the runner, dealing in generalities that toe the party lines to accommodate their common non-athletic constituents. Being a runner then requires me to take an active interest in my body fuel, which drives my performance capability beyond the general population's needs. While I don't have special metabolic requirements, I did realize early in life garbage in equates to garbage out! And by "*out*," I mean my health and enjoyment of running.

So, when it comes to fuel for my body, I adopt a few simple rules for what goes in my mouth based on my own experience on how my body has reacted to it in the past and how it makes me feel. We've all experienced the foods that pull your stomach down to your knees the morning after. Worse are the ones that explode in your gut in mid-run, requiring a pitstop in full view of nature. These lessons are learned quickly.

We're "*food and drink*" consumers caught between our conditioned tastes, and the fact is, satisfying those preferences is poisoning our bodies. Anybody involved in serious shopping at a supermarket knows the score. It's a battle between the food giants whose aim is to make you buy more of their stuff using literally "*sweetened*" deals. Sugar addiction is real, and almost anything in a box or can is not directly from nature. I decided a while ago to be a conscientious objector in that war. I play a game once a week where I count how many aisles I go down. Less is more and better, given the aisles are littered with processed foods.

I don't subscribe to any particular diet, but I lean toward protein and vegetables as it keeps purchases and preparation simple and helps with weight maintenance. I enjoy salads, seafood, most meat, dairy, and enjoy baking. I limit my intake of foods and drink rich and soaked in calories but can be tempted once in a while. I stopped taking sugar in any beverages passing my lips many years ago. Our household consumes a lot of organic fruit during the week, and I have a banana most days before my run. I read about the latest fad diets but understand not every diet is proper or works for every person, so don't force your square peg body into a round hole diet. Most diets are invented in books written by medical doctors who don't run, so be skeptical. You choose what's suitable for your body and activity level. Each of us has a relationship with food that's emotional and thereby complicated.

I wasn't that into food growing up in England. We certainly didn't have the selection of processed foods available today. Still, growing up in a family on a diet of meat and potatoes, I didn't pay much attention to any significance over what went in my mouth and my body.

I was able to do my training and didn't seem to suffer health-wise. I've always had a sweet tooth and still do today, but nowadays, I curb this tendency, whereas back in my early running days, a dose of refined sugar snacks as part of my daily food intake wasn't uncommon. Without watching my diet and food types, I always got a healthy diagnosis at my annual checkups. Although the blood tests identified I'd bad cholesterol levels as I got older, I always had outstanding numbers of the good cholesterol level. So my physician never lectured me about paying more attention to my food diet.

However, this has changed in the last few decades, and I've uncovered some truths about food and me. My cholesterol got out of balance, so I can no longer ignore experimenting on what makes a healthy diet for me. In so doing, I've discovered a taste for vegetables, and I'm living proof you can learn to love vegetables. For some inexplicable reason, Smoothies send me to the hospital with embarrassing gastronomical issues that nobody understands. Organic foods, in most instances, are better for me.

When it comes to vitamins, I take a few. One of the doctors in my journey (they do seem to come in and out of my life frequently) prescribed Vitamin D3, and there seems general medical agreement this is appropriate at my age. My annual checkup blood testing has not turned up any other deficiencies requiring additional vitamins. However, because I run, I also take vitamin C supplements, as runners commonly advocate for this. But you should attend regular checkups and blood tests as a runner to uncover any lurking issues.

The essential choice for you to make is a doctor who runs. I don't take advice on my running from friends who don't run, so why would I take advice from a doctor who doesn't run? Doctors who run may be a rare breed, but they exist, and you'll need to insist. Most doctors, after all, would prefer you didn't run as it's hazardous to your body, which is an inaccurate blanket statement.

When it comes to fluids, I don't regularly drink alcohol, preferring water or flavored spring water. I appreciate an occasional glass of wine, but I'm not into a beer of any kind these days. As a runner, I need to worry about hydration and making sure I replenish throughout the day after my workout run, and water is my best friend to achieve this.

I do enjoy coffee but limit my intake to two cups a day in the morning. I may take a decaf coffee in the afternoon or evening in rare instances, but it's unusual, and I prefer tea in the afternoon or relaxing late in the day.

I make every attempt to put good fuel in my body but also don't ignore festivities where baking is on the menu for the day. The next day's run may remind me why I should've abstained from the cake, but as I plod through the first miles and feel recovery, I don't let the guilt linger even when the stomach suggests otherwise. I also eat as much organically grown food as I can to avoid pesticides, especially fruit which has an essential role in my diet. I realize there's a cost element and a decision for folks—organics are more expensive and a sorry statement on our food industry.

Being a runner, I'm always concerned about maintaining a healthy body so I can do the things I enjoy... *like running*. Because my lower joints are an essential part of my body equipment, one thing that can stop me from enjoying my running is inflammation. We know certain foods and how they're processed can cause inflammation in the body. This is different from inflammation caused by my exercise, which is part of the natural healing process. We know chronic inflammation can be triggered by a diet high in refined sugars and carbohydrates and an abundance of dairy. So, while these foods are not absent entirely from my diet, there's a conscious effort to limit my exposure to their harmful effects. If you're tuned to *"listening to your body,"* then the limit for you will echo in how you feel, particularly in your gut. Bloated and feeling listless are real and symptoms your diet may need adjusting.

Portions is another topic altogether. My first few years in America were a significant adjustment in the amount of food classed as a standard serving with friends at home or in a restaurant. Back in the 1980s, it was a wide-eyed shock to Europeans and me and those from the Far East even today regarding the oversized portions served up in America. We even bought special plates for use at home for the family to reduce our portion sizes. The simple adage stop when you feel full, though sound advice, does require you to eat slower, so you give your brain the time to catch up with your stomach to trigger your "*full*" message.

I'm a three-meals-a-day person but only eat when I'm hungry, and my meals can be some other runner's version of a lite snack. I'm not a big person, fluctuating on either side of the dial of 130lbs, and with a small frame, my daily calorie intake is adjusted to my size and activity level. I avoid snacks during the day unless I'm hungry and avoid food habits that have nothing to do with being hungry. That all being said, I do allow myself the occasional day off from the healthy diet grid. At the very least, the after-body effects of these beautiful gastronomical excursions remind me of why it's infrequent.

I don't find that running impacts my appetite like other runners report. So, I can eat my breakfast within 30 minutes of my workout or go for long periods before and after my run before hunger visits me. In our household, we do our best to eat dinner as a family to catch up with each other; it also makes us feel like a community. You'll need to find what works for you, but your running will dictate your meals moving forward or the other way around, depending on your circumstances. Find a routine that works for you and others you live with and stay with it. Having habits around food is good for harmony in a household.

Have many meals in your repertoire that provide good fuel for you and whomever else you're cooking for regularly. This lets you plan out the week and your grocery shopping ahead of time. Keep it predominately simple and easy to prepare. Include some baking recipes that have relatively healthy ingredients and include less or substitute refined sugars. I'm no chef and only passable as a cook compared to my spouse's years of experience, but the last few years of juggling food chores and running have required some adjustments in my kitchen habits and skills.

Also, take your time to enjoy your food. We don't seem to delight in our food anymore. It's become an activity we have to get done as quickly as possible so we can get on to... what? TV or reading, relaxing or back to work? In our house, dinner is mostly the only time we all get together. No talking at the table isn't part of our modus operandi either, as it also helps slow our speed of eating and digestion. Another reason is to repeat my earlier thought about providing your brain the opportunity to catch up with your stomach so you get the signals you're full and don't need any more fuel.

I already mentioned my preference for water over other fluids. I'm prone to leg and foot cramps, especially in the hours after a long run, and this is because I don't pay as much attention to hydration as I should, especially at my age. If this is you also, but you've better hydration habits than me, there may be something else needing to be corrected, and a blood check through your doctor will help pinpoint it or at least put your mind at rest. In the past, I've done the drinking fluids quantity according to my bodyweight routine a few times in my life, but it always ends up with too much of my time focused on bladder management.

I feel the weight and water intake calculations are not accurate, at least for me, and going to pee the number of times required for comfort was just washing away all the good nutrients in my body. Finding the sweet spot for your weight requires experimentation to manage appropriately what you put in and not lead to bloating or finding the location for your next restroom trip.

I believe eating and drinking healthy comes down to common sense and habits. Common sense is that most mature adults know what's good and what isn't to put in our bodies. Bad habits form because we struggle when it comes to making the right choices on an ongoing basis. There are plenty of obese and overweight people who know more about food and diets than I'll ever know. They're hoping to find a diet that lets them eat the foods they love and be their right size. Running can be a part of their born-again body and enjoying life, but it still requires nourishing fuel to get and keep you there.

For more information around changing habits and making them stick, see the resource section at the companion website to this book here: www.RunToEnjoyLife.com

So, we've covered a lot here, but hopefully, I won't be pulled to pieces by any doctors or textbook nutritionists advocating specific diets not approved by the academy of whatever. Just remember you're a runner, and you're an experiment of one, so do your research and investigation and always be skeptical regardless of how many letters after their name. When it comes to diets, even the doctors can't seem to agree.

Next up, we talk about running routes and schedules and some other habits to make our running and life more enjoyable.

CHAPTER TWELVE

Mapping Out Your World

"Difficult roads often lead to beautiful destinations"
– Attributed to Zig Ziglar

To truly enjoy my runs, I must be outdoors on roads or trails winding around Cape Cod's lakes and ponds or along the coast on Falmouth Heights and Vineyard Sound. It's in these places I feel the freedom and quietness of my own feet and breath and thoughts.

I choose my running routes as carefully as I would in renting an apartment or buying a house. I have my criteria it must meet. It must be a good loop length. Include some hills to tackle to break up the rhythm, woods, and water that attract birds and animal sounds, color, fragrance, and quiet roads free of noise and constant traffic. But mostly, I need a feeling of calm and harmony from familiarity, knowing what to expect, and not interrupting surprises.

Of course, this is a utopia, and unreasonable you may think for you, especially if you live in an urban rather than a rural area. Or a long way from water or forests. But wherever you carry out your runs, you'll plan and add variety as best you can for your routes, schedule your workouts taking into account rest days and the impact all this has on your safety and performance. There are links between all of these, as you'll see.

This chapter will share what works for me and my thoughts on putting together your routes on the path to your own Everest and achieving your other goals, all while enjoying the journey.

I've touched on some of these topics in earlier chapters, but I'll repeat some material in a different context for you, which will help emphasize the points.

Choosing your routes where you'll run should be done carefully. I prefer routes that take me along quiet roads and have small loops of around 5-6 miles. I've got a few in my repertoire chosen for variety and catering for different types of runs. Alternating between different routes and surfaces keeps your workouts interesting. You may find a route and stay with it, rarely needing a change and preferring familiarity over variety.

Busy roads are a safety concern for runners. Drivers are not always paying attention or expect to be sharing the road with a runner. They're often distracted listening to the radio or music on their MP3 or trying to follow map directions. Worse, they may be in conversation on the phone. You get the picture—they're distracted for many different reasons and not seeing you running in the road toward them.

Another reason for choosing quiet roads is that once you get out of residential areas, there may be no sidewalk to run on, and you're forced to run on the road itself. Even in the residential area where I live, there are little to no sidewalks. Certainly, busy roads and highways have no sidewalk, so runners are forced to run in the street gutter with all the debris and drains and unevenness associated with that area of the road.

When choosing a route, look for ones that take you along or around ponds or lakes and parks and wooded areas. These areas attract wildlife which adds pleasant sounds to your run and provides scenery breaks. The point is to choose routes that are enjoyable to run along for most of the time. Depending on where you live, you may be forced to run on a busy road or highway for some of the time—I have one such route—but plan to minimize how long you're on that particular road. Additionally, cut down on interruptions on your route. If you can avoid intersections, especially with traffic lights, do so. They interrupt your flow and enjoyment, and of course, force a break when you may be doing a time trial.

As I mentioned, I prefer loops of 5 – 6 miles for my running. I don't want to be any further than 2 – 3 miles from home if an injury or other event happens. I want to be able to walk home if possible. Having a short circuit for your run also provides you the capability of taking care of toilet concerns. Being caught short out on a run can lead to embarrassing situations. I make a point of emptying myself in the bathroom before I go out. Before a race due to nervous energy, this can require a few visits. I like to be comfortable running, and needing to go to the bathroom mid-way through your run or miles from home puts you in a bind and focused on something else and not enjoying your run. If possible, plan your routes so there are places where you can go to the bathroom in an emergency and away from public view.

When you start, and you're just running for 15 – 20 minutes, your routes may be shorter than mine. 1 – 2 miles is okay—I used to run along a 1½ mile route which wasn't a loop but out and back, and you can certainly do this for your beginning routes. Instead of loops, you have out and back for a total of 3 – 6 miles. Same difference as loops.

I like loops because I can do a longer run using them if my schedule calls for it. So, my long run on a Sunday of 12 –15 miles is two loops of one of my routes. It keeps the run more enjoyable, whereas out and backs mean I'm running on the same roads for hours, which can become tedious. You decide on what makes sense for you.

Know your mile markers along the routes you choose as well. I like to know how my run and how my pace is going, and if you don't have a GPS watch, then a viable alternative is to time your markers, so you've got a sense of how your run is going. If I intend to do a faster run along my route but find I'm struggling with a decent pace at mile one or two, then I know this may not be a good day for a fast run—aka listening to my body—so I can ease off and save it for the next workout.

I like to have a sense of my next week's running schedule to prepare other activities around them. I'm not paranoid about it, just working out what days will be rest days and what days are easy runs or more strenuous interval sessions—fast repeats, etc. I aim for a minimum of 40 miles per week, having worked up to that mileage over a few years since I started back up seriously. For you, if you're beginning, you may be running on time in shoes than miles. This is fine. Still, keep a log of miles run each session and total for the week, even if it seems small to you at 5 or 10 miles. Recording your mileage also doubles as triggering when to replace your running shoes.

Suppose one of your goals is to complete a marathon in a specific time. In that case, many recommend a base of 30 miles per week for a year before tackling a 16-week program to complete a marathon in 4 or 41/2 hours and avoid injury or placing stress on your body before it's ready. If you're not running to break a specific time and just to finish, then providing you can complete a 20-mile session a few times before the race, then likely you can finish one. See my marathon section in the additional materials at the end of the book for more.

When you do your running is usually based on work and family commitments and personal preference. For me, this has been adjusted through the years, and while your body can adapt to almost exercise at any time, I now prefer to do mine early morning when it's light outside, so I'm easily visible on the roads. I've run in the dark on well-lit streets when a youth, but now there's too much at risk of injury on roads where drivers can't see me, and I can't see what my feet are going to be stepping on next.

However, running after dusk or before dawn may be the only time available to you. If so, then look for routes that are well lit. This may be easier to do in urban areas than in rural areas where street lighting is not a town priority. You can also purchase head or belt lamps for night running that not only help you light up the road but make you more easily visible to vehicle drivers.

I had spells in my life when I ran after work, when I got home, and before dinner. This can work for you and gives you some "*me*" time before settling down with the family and after the drain of the workday is over. It can release stress and provide a bridge between work and family time. But I found this didn't work for me during the winter months and forced me to run on a treadmill or at a gym more, and this extra time in my day made me unavailable to the family until long after work had finished. If you're beyond these worries, and especially during the warmer months, running in the evening during daylight can have a calming effect on you and your thoughts during the hours of the day before final relaxation.

So, you're going to choose when you run based on your circumstances and situations, which could change throughout the week. I'm certainly not obsessed with having to run first thing in the morning. I adjust if the weather is foul but is forecasted to improve later, or if it's cold but will warm up by waiting a few hours. Again, I've got that luxury, but you may not.

If you're an individual who prefers to run with others, finding different routes will likely be part of your game plan anyway. My current running club in Falmouth has a 5-mile run at 5:30 pm every Friday for all-comers, even non-members and vacation visitors. It's run throughout the year, but I take a break from it during the winter months. You can make it as competitive or not as the mood takes you. It's a scenic 5-mile route with some coastline and quiet roads. It allows me to run in a group at a leisurely pace or push myself on other occasions at near race pace. Joining a running club offers opportunities to try new routes with other runners and feel even more part of a community. I strongly advise it.

As a final component of all this, I want to discuss your running performance related to your schedule.

Never lose sight of why you're running. You're running to enjoy yourself. A desire to run was likely stimulated initially by getting fit, keeping healthy, and feeling better about yourself. There is a myriad of schedules out there for all levels and goals. If you need help in choosing a program that can work for you and your goals, then you'll find some resources at the companion website to this book here: www.RunToEnjoyLife.com

For new runners, then your goal may be a 5k or 10k race. Or a run for a fun one-mile race. Your goal may be just completing a 5k run as opposed to running a specific time. Looking at a selection of training schedules can absorb you for several research hours. There may be several false starts and switching of schedules before finding one that fits your capabilities and lifestyle and keeps you interested and improving. The point is what works for one runner may not work for you, and this is okay. The schedule, and you, need to be flexible and adjust. Rigidity is the cause of boredom, lack of enjoyment, and stagnates performance improvement.

We all want to see improvement in our running. Even if we're mainly running for enjoyment, we still wish to experience visible gains from our time investment. This can take many forms. Improvement in heart rate at rest, more energy and less tired in our day, sleeping well at night. But it's valid to want improvement in how long we can run for and at what pace. This is only natural as it indicates we're on the right path. This is especially true when preparing for a distance race. The schedule you have will have milestones and pace times for your training, and if you're not capable of *"keeping pace"* with the schedule, it just means your body isn't ready yet. So, lower your sights. Being realistic with yourself not only avoids disappointment, which you get over quickly once you're back on the road but, more importantly, reduces the chance of injury.

I've also found over the years that runners reach a plateau and improve in *"fits and starts."* This has happened with me, and I've seen it in many others. I had a runner friend who was stuck at a 5:30-minute mile pace over 5-mile road races for a long time even though his training schedule suggested he should be able to race 5-minute mile pace. He didn't waver from his program but kept at it. One day, he ran a 5-mile race at a 5-minute mile pace and subsequently surpassed that result. He had reached a plateau and, for some time, just went along with the schedule and then burst through.

So, don't be discouraged if you reach a stage where you seem stuck. Indeed, there are ways to get out of being stuck—change of training schedule, workout partners—new routes. But my point here is to expect it and focus on enjoyment in your running and not to measure that enjoyment by performance only. If you do, it'll break your heart all the time. If you put in the time and effort, you'll get the results just like in life.

So, we covered a lot in this chapter around choosing routes and a schedule that'll work for you and get you outdoors running regularly and enjoying life, and what to expect for all this activity you're pouring yourself into.

The next chapter will focus on your overall perspective and habits, how to ensure you're running isn't at the expense of everything else, and how habits can help in all these areas.

CHAPTER THIRTEEN

Keeping Everything in Perspective

"Nothing happens to you, it happens for you.
See the positive in negative events."
– Joel Osteen

Running is an essential part of who I am and my identity, but it isn't my whole life.

While I love my running for all the reasons I've discussed in earlier chapters, it's not what drives me to get up each day.

Running is there if I choose to use it, but it's there the next day if I don't. It doesn't desert me or feel neglected or hurt if I decide not to run one day or take a more extended break. It's not a complicated relationship needing constant love and attention. I can leave it out of my life for a while—as I have—but it always welcomes me back when I decide to pick up my shoes, slip them on, and pound the roads again.

None of this means I don't take my running seriously or treat my body with respect. Exercise should be a part of our life. I choose running. Compared to *"early man,"* we live sedentary lives, which in a weird twist of fate makes us more vulnerable to risks... of the health kind. Our ancient ancestors had to keep moving to stay alive. In many respects, this requirement is even more needed today. Movement is key to our health and life. For me, this isn't only about physical movement but mental progression as well. It's only through progression in all its forms that we can achieve our goals and be all we can be.

Goals help our movement. Goals are for our life. They should be more than fitness goals. Fitness goals are so you get healthy enough to achieve everything else you want out of your life.

I've embraced running in my life but not as an obsession at the expense of everything else. It took me some time to find the balance and look at running as a friend I can visit whenever I want but not use it as a replacement for life.

Running has introduced me to many relationships. People who run, I've generally found, provide excellent company. Running in a group is a way to get out and enjoy the day. I had such a particular group many years ago when young. They were mostly older men than I, and they took me under their wing. Their pace was mainly leisurely, but this allowed for plenty of chatter, and they talked about things that, at my young age, I couldn't always relate to. But it was good of them to allow me to be running in their pack and be treated as an equal.

But there are times when running alone provides the quietness for thought and connection with the natural world. I'm mostly okay with my own company. I'm an introvert. But that doesn't mean to say I'm lonely. I've never felt lonely. I enjoy the company of others. I enjoy being with my family and doing things with them and experiencing their lives and celebrating their successes, and supporting them as they grow. They teach me lessons every day still. When I worked in the corporate world, the relationships I forged helped me make it through the more challenging days at work or home.

But if I'm left at the end of the day with time alone, this is also a form of enjoyment. We all need to be alone and have time to ourselves on occasions—even the extroverts among us.

Runners come in all shapes, sizes, temperaments, and habits. We all have habits. If you remember, I mentioned I'd learned many years ago, how you do anything is how you do everything. This is true about running and life and our habits.

If you're consistent about your running, you'll likely be consistent about other aspects of your life. If you procrastinate or easily brush off your workout as the mood takes you, then this mindset will manifest itself elsewhere in your life. How we approach small things mirrors our attitude to essential things in our life. If all your runs are easy on level terrain with no challenges, does this echo your life? Do you find the familiarity of always choosing the same route safe and calming and no need to experiment and take other paths? Do you look at your running as an opportunity to play or put on your fight face when you tie your shoes? The lessons we learn through running can be applied in our life outside running.

There should be no judgment on how you answer the above questions. There's no right or wrong. Just the way it is for you. If you want to change aspects of your life, then start with your running. Running can provide a healing environment for you and a personal lab to experiment with habit changes and see how they work to take into the rest of your life.

What are my primary habits for running, and more importantly, how do I feel they're reflected in my life? I'll take a shot at some realistic self-analysis, knowing that a psychologist could probably have a field day with all this and offer up some insights different from mine. But at the end of the day, we make the hard life-change decisions ourselves.

Here are my top 5 running habits...

1. **I run 4 – 6 days a week, at least for one hour per day throughout the year.**
2. **I run outdoors.**
3. **I listen to my body.**
4. **I stretch to prepare.**
5. **I buy new running shoes every 500 – 750 miles.**

Let's look at each one and what I believe it says about me. You may dismiss these or not agree with any of these habits, and this is okay. You'll find your habits and reasons, but just make sure you reflect on what they say about you. And if you feel your running habits are out of sync with the rest of your life, then make changes.

I run 4 – 6 days a week at least one hour per day throughout the year:

This is primarily about being realistic with myself. I decided that I would adopt a schedule my life could sustain the last time I started running again. I didn't want to have something to aim for that would take years to get to but something I could achieve quickly. I've worked up to 4 – 6 days and had a lower target at the beginning. If you're starting, you may want to aim for running 10 – 20 minutes three times a week until you feel ready to increase either length of session or frequency.

Some weeks I've done more as regards sessions or time running. This is especially true when preparing for a long race such as a ½ or full marathon. But I've never fallen below the minimum of 4 days of one-hour runs in a week for the last three years. Some weeks it's been challenging to do due to work or personal stuff going on. That's life. But keeping a realistic minimum is vital to ensure I get that success feeling in my life.

Being successful in this habit spills over into my life. I set realistic minimums in other areas now and rarely disappoint myself with my effort. This is different from all those years of scheduling a list of twenty things to do in a day and getting to about 3 or 4 of them. This not only makes you feel like you didn't achieve anything, but it exhausts you! You beat yourself up and slip into negative self-talk, which can quickly become a habit in other aspects of your life.

I'm not afraid to say *"no"* to an ask for my time. When looking at my life schedule for the week and detailing my running schedule, some adjustments may need to be made to keep them in sync. This is okay, as I know there's power in the word *'no."*

I Run Outdoors:

My second habit is to run outdoors. This I do for most workouts. But I'm also not obsessed about it if I can't get outdoors. The weather doesn't always allow me. In New England, the winters work against you some days, so the treadmill is my backup.

I don't mind running in rain, providing it's not a heavy downpour, and usually, I can wait for an hour or two for it to lessen or subside. But snow and ice are not road conditions I'm willing to put myself at risk to do for the sake of my preferred terrain. So, if I want to run that day, then I'm okay running on a treadmill. I find running on a treadmill hard. You'd think that running an 8-minute mile on a treadmill would be easier given you're propelled along by a machine, but not me. I find running 8-minute or 9-minute miles comes easier outdoors. But as much as I prefer the outdoors, I'm willing to adjust my habit as circumstances dictate rather than being foolhardy about it and risking injury to my body.

Life is like this as well. You may have a habit you feel must be done in a certain way at all costs. Some folks may think that if they don't stick to it and adjust, their whole life will break down, and their spouse will leave them, and their kids will never love them again, and they'll end up murdered in a deserted alley! Yes, I know it's ridiculous, but we do makeup stores like this, and sometimes taking it to the extreme makes you realize how stupid defending a habit can be if it's not serving you any longer.

Adjusting your habit to see another day won't cause the collapse of your Roman Empire.

I Listen to My Body:

Pay attention to what your body is telling you. Assuming you're not always looking for an excuse to avoid exercising if your body is telling you today isn't a good day to run, don't. Walk instead or do some other activity; as I've mentioned before, you can even start running and decide to cut it short or stop and resort to walking home. You've many options.

On the other hand, if your body is telling you today is a good day, and you can adjust the session you were going to do, performing speed interval work instead, or even a tempo workout in place of an easy run, then go for it.

The point here is to get into the habit of listening to your body, and you'll recognize these opportunities. It's a great feeling to start out thinking one way and then change your mind because of what your body is feeling that day. It exercises your "*flexibility*" muscle and provides an important feedback loop for you. And yes, I've just drifted from running into the impact "*listening*" has on my personal life. Now listening in this context includes your mind and body. The act of listening to your mind is every bit as necessary.

Some of you reading this may struggle with the concept of listening to your body and mind, especially in the sense of your everyday life. What does it mean, and how does it work and feel practically?

For me, I've noticed an improvement in my ability to cope with change, particularly in stressful situations. Experts tell us our mind thinks around 2,100 thoughts per hour, and our thoughts lead to our feelings. You've just had a bunch of thoughts in the few seconds it took you to read these sentences. So, when I'm under stress, I've racing thoughts, and some of them not particularly helpful, so I acknowledge these thoughts and let them pass through and move on without acting on them or allowing them to affect how I feel. They are, after all, just thoughts and only as real as I choose to make them.

Listening to my body and how I'm feeling prepares me for listening to my mind and its thoughts and processing these thoughts for richer or poorer in my life. I get to decide what to act on or not. Thoughts, feelings, and actions lead to results. It's all interconnected, and for me, making better choices has been instrumental in enjoying my life more.

I Stretch to Prepare:

I have a bunch of stretching exercises I do before and after my run. I've been stretching before my running all my life. Now, the exercises have changed as I've gotten older and adjusted for my body weaknesses, but I've always stretched. It just seems the right thing to do for me. It also not only gets my physical body ready for running but also prepares me mentally.

It also provides a first check-in opportunity before I run on how my body is feeling today. How am I for stiffness and aches? Am I recovered from my last run? Is there tightness I haven't felt before? You get the drift.

My stretches primarily focus on the lower body and leg muscles and groin area, which seems to be my historically weak points. I don't want to get into the whole debate about whether stretching prevents injuries or not; as for me, it's irrelevant. I stretch before and after a run, and I've encountered relatively few injuries in my years compared to most other runners I know. It just makes sense to me and takes 5-minutes before and after.

I practice prepping and mental stretching in my life. I think we all do to a certain extent. Any of this sound familiar? Making sure your seat belt is secure, and you're looking in all the mirrors for other cars before making a maneuver. Mapping out a route to somewhere, so you arrive on time. Planning and scheduling so you don't forget an important event. Preparing for an exam, so you feel ready to do your best. These are all just forms of stretching, both physical and mental.

I Buy New Running Shoes Every 750 Miles:

I can hear you… where is he going with this habit?

Well, this one is all about throwing out the old (sneakers) and bringing in the new (*shining clean with go-faster stripes*) sneakers when they still may have mileage on them. Said that way, this may seem like an extravagant habit to have, but I ignored it for so long, and for me, at my age, it provides me peace of mind. I'm doing what I feel is right to protect my body.

Again, I've covered this in my chapter on equipment. Having good support between me and the road is critical for my well-being. Running shoes take a beating and not something I skimp on, as it's my primary protection when running. It's the most expensive item on my budget but worth every penny I pay.

As I've increased my weekly mileage, I replace my shoes quicker than I did a few years ago, translating into increased costs. Some shoes also break down faster than others, requiring me to change more frequently. I just don't rely on miles run in a pair, but what my body is telling me. I know by the feeling of my muscles and joints when it's time to change and do so quickly.

Like most runners, your shoes do get a second life as casual sneakers. They still have some mileage left in them for walking or doing errands. You'll soon accumulate a rack of second-life sneakers, and your family will ask awkward questions about why you have so many. Tell them to deal with it.

This habit of a pre-emptive strike has slipped quietly into my life as well. I just don't put up with things around the house, or in my life, not working, or past their prime, any longer. I used to be that type of person who didn't want to spend the money, or I would put up with something not working because I was in the *"I'll wait until it irritates me"* mode before resolving. We make an emotional decision and then justify it with our logic... even when it's flawed logic.

Now there are other habits I have in my running that I'd deem as insignificant. They're more like routines, but I do them in a specific order because they're my habits. I always put my gear on in a particular order and do my stretches in a specific sequence. But the above five I view as significant as they spill over into my life. You'll determine your running habits and how you implement them into your life. It'll happen naturally, so I wouldn't overthink it too much.

I began this chapter on how I keep my running in perspective and shared my habits to emphasize that perspective and my examples. Of course, your lessons and habits will reflect your own experiences, but my premise here has been to encourage you to make it a healthy perspective. It's easy to slip into making running your whole life, but I think that would be a mistake, and you'll miss out on the wider enjoyment of life.

In the next chapter, I want to put everything together for you in one place. It'll be somewhat of a recap for you but a place you can return to and refresh as you see relevant during the exciting months and years that lay ahead for you.

CHAPTER FOURTEEN

Putting It All Together

*"Age is just a state of mind but sometimes
the mind gets in a state!"*
– Richard Calderwood

In running world terms, I'm beginning to wind down here. We've almost finished the journey I started with you, and now it's time for me to ease off the pace. This section then will take each of the various lessons I've learned in my more than five decades of running and shared in the previous chapters and make it real for you in your everyday life. Think of it as a quick reference to refresh and remind yourself of all the ways you can add enjoyment to your running and life.

Your life situation may be different from mine. Your goals and desires may be dissimilar as well. And so, how you use the information I've shared will necessarily be part of your analysis and implementation. This way, you'll also take ownership of what you decide to change and enhance.

We are quick to blame others or circumstances when things don't work out as we plan. It's easy to slip into the victim mentality. But at the end of the day, it's up to us and how we choose to think and feel about an outcome—expected or unexpected. We can let any training run or race make a good day or form the foundation of a disappointing one. We choose our thoughts and, thereby, how we feel.

Here is a recap of my strategies with more reinforcement and suggestions for you, so you have more good days than disappointing ones.

1.   Listening to Your Body and Mind:

A common thread throughout my life has been about listening to my body and mind and what it's telling me. It isn't as difficult as you may think. It's not about being the right brain instead of the left brain. It's logical and doesn't require any creative genius in you. What we aren't so good at is deliberately taking notice of what we're feeling or experiencing and acting on it. We're dismissive of it, or worse, ignore it entirely and soldier on hoping things will get better. But it rarely does.

If I get pain in my knee beyond normal twitches or just stiffness when I'm out running, and it persists, it may force me to stop running and reconsider if today is a good day to run? It doesn't mean I can't run tomorrow because my knee is acting up today, just a situation requiring me to save myself for another day, to wait until it's healed. My body has told me to stop, or at least not to run today.

This is the same in life. What's your body and mind telling you as you go about your personal and family life? Are you ignoring its signs and how you feel? Are you dismissive about your own needs and consider them subservient to others? Do you let yourself become the victim of not listening because you fall into the common trap of putting other's needs before your own?

After all, remember the flight attendant's pre-flight talk about in the event of an emergency, and the oxygen mask comes down to put your own on first before you help others with theirs. So don't be afraid to do it. Attend to your needs first to provide better attention to others, be it family, friends, colleagues at work, or where you volunteer.

You now know listening to your body and mind and acting on what you feel and what it's telling you is one of the essential deeds you can do for your running and well-being.

2. Major and Minor Props:

All you need is a desire and a pair of excellent supportive running shoes to go out running. Everything else is just an accessory. There are lots of other gear you could purchase to make yourself more comfortable, but I've never found any of these to make my running more *"enjoyable."* Just more convenient. As my running shoes are my primary aid and protection for my body to achieve the health and fitness I want in my life, I pay particular attention to those shoes' quality—no skimping or cutting corners to get the best support for my feet I can.

This mirrors life as well. You could have plenty of accessories in your life, but what is the equivalent of your *"running shoes?"* Is it your family? Or your career? Or a community? We each get to choose what we consider is essential in our life. Some people have goals to help them in their life journey and invest their time and money in achieving their aims. This is healthy.

In my own life, my family comes first in my today and my future. It's like the sole of my running shoes.

Make sure you've got an excellent pair of running shoes to focus on enjoying your running, and likewise attend to your own basic needs so you can enjoy your own life and those you care about. Keep things simple and basic. If you get the basics in running right, then you'll have the energy and focus on being the best you can be in your life.

3. The Power of Play:

Keeping spark in our lives can sometimes mean allowing in plenty of fun and room for being playful. I don't mean being flippant about your running or life but merely saying it's okay to spice things up to keep it interesting.

My running could become tedious if I let it. The same route, terrain, and pace every day don't let me improve and grow in my running. I've long-term goals for my running and in my personal life. And as my running and life is a journey, these challenges will change. Either because I'll achieve what I want or because my circumstances change over time. What mattered a few years ago isn't as important any longer. Life has a way of throwing up challenges that make you rethink your destinations and how you want them to look.

But none of this changes the need to enjoy life by including play in it in the present. If you find your work fun and it adds variety and interest to your life, this is fine and shouldn't make you feel guilty. But I've generally found that having other interests outside work can provide relaxation and a sense of fulfillment in our life that we all need.

Sometimes we have to "*work*" at introducing play into our life. As strange as this sounds, this is common. It's easy to get to a point where we don't know how to have fun any longer. This can be especially true when we're under financial stress, and the only way out of this seems to be to work harder to get more income. Life then becomes a treadmill—and you already know how I feel about treadmills.

So, schedule in play in your running and life. Pay attention to this to avoid getting stale and letting negative thoughts overtake you.

4. Paying Attention and Avoiding Distractions:

You can see how many things in life are connected, but it's easy to lose sight of these links. When you're running outdoors, remember the reasons why you're in that place at that time; to rediscover nature and enjoy surroundings and the spirit of freedom it imparts on you. You aren't just there to perform a workout but to get into the flow, prepare for the day, or experience healing. Do this by focusing on your surroundings to experience the run. Avoid any distractions that take away from your experience. Leave the earbuds at home so you can pay attention to the present and the road ahead.

Know where your feet will land next and see the road ahead, so you avoid obstacles and anticipate threats when sharing the road with vehicles. I prefer to be in control of my running rather than leaving it to others or fate.

Life is the same. Pay attention to the important things and avoid wasteful distractions that consume your time with no return. The distractions I'm talking about are those different from play and having fun, for these provide recreation and rejuvenation for your body and mind. Wasteful distractions in your life are doing things that take you off course or cause you to lose focus or completing the task at hand. They stop you from keeping the promises you've made to yourself.

5. Rainy Mornings and Sunny Afternoons:

Regardless of when you do your running for the day, it allows you to restart the day. To reset an unproductive or draining *"before"* to a productive and reenergized *"after."* Take what I call *"rainy mornings"* and turn them into *"sunny afternoons,"* at least metaphorically speaking.

My running session is usually done early morning, so it doesn't split my day into two equal halves. In fact, sometimes, I don't have a chance to have a *"challenging morning"* before my run.

Nonetheless, it's still an opportunity to set a positive tone for the day ahead. On your running day, you may run at lunchtime or after work. In either instance, you can let your run split your day up and get a second chance of having a great remainder of the day with a positive attitude after a pleasant workout.

How does this translate into your life?

Well, in many respects, the mere act of running can set you in the right mood for what remains of your day—a chance to replace any dampening of spirits caused by events before your workout. Experience informs us that when a project or activity isn't going well, keeping at it until it gets better can work against us. We need to stop and pull back and have a change of pace or activity. This is designed to take our mind off something that's causing a negative loop in our brain. You can also think of it as a disaster movie continuously playing in our head that isn't getting us to where we want to be or causing us stress. If things don't change, they remain the same no matter how many times we repeat the movie.

So, stack the odds in your favor for enjoying life by introducing activities to change course from a bad day to a good day. Do something else if you can. Introduce play or fun during your break.

Not every day can be entirely enjoyable, but where it ends up in your mind is all up to you and your thoughts and where you decide to take it. Just don't accept you can't change it. Resignation to the way your day is going and "*pulling the covers over your head*" gives up control to your current thoughts and feelings, which, if not positive, you can reverse and thereby end up in a different place than you would've otherwise.

6. Reducing and Recovering from Injuries:

Understand that you'll get injuries at some point. The hope is that they're minor and keep you out for just a few days or weeks.

Pounding the pavement or trails, no matter how many miles you do, eventually, you'll find your leg muscles and joints will revolt back at you and demand some rest. This is just the nature of running.

Also, accidents happen. A misplaced foot here or there or a slip or unexpected fall can cause ankle sprains and muscle tears. An awkward winter slip on ice can even cause a head injury and concussion.

Reducing injuries becomes then cutting your odds down of having one. A comfortable, good quality pair of running shoes to give you support and replacing them frequently on a mileage schedule helps, as does paying attention when you're out and avoiding distractions. As I've repeated in different contexts, know where your next step will be and what is there. Making good choices about the conditions you run in and where you run are additional factors in helping to keep you free of injury.

These precautions also spill over into life and factor in how we treat our health and relationships, which all add to the enjoyment of our life. While I'm not suggesting you reduce adventures in your life and be paranoid and become overly risk-averse, just understand your risk tolerance based on your own life experiences. The level of risk you take will generally change as you age, and thoughts of your mortality impact your decisions.

I've talked about taking time and not rushing to get back on the road or track to train on recovering from injuries. If an injury occurs or comes on when you're out running, walk home if you can. If you can't, then seek help. Carry your phone with you so you can get a ride. Let your body heal and take care of it. Seek professional help if needed to aid recovery.

Sprains and muscle injuries can take weeks to recover and can be frustrating but be gentle on your body and mind. You'll recover with care and attention and time. It can be incredibly disappointing to lose two or six weeks of training for a marathon or half-marathon. But better to take the stress off yourself and live to run another race than cause a significant injury to your body that affects not only your running ability but walking and gait permanently.

The body is an amazing device if left to heal itself naturally. This is also true in life, as our body is our vehicle through life, and we only get one in our lifetime, so take care of it.

7. Avoiding "Burnout" but Keeping the Edge:

Have a realistic training schedule, especially if you're preparing for a particular race. But it's also okay to not have a major plan or race and just get out each day to enjoy your run and be in the outdoors. Have a routine that supports your enjoyment. Running hard every day is a recipe for getting stale and injured quickly, so make time for easy runs, whether it's most days or all days.

Find ways of keeping the adventure and interest there, though—what I call keeping an "*edge.*" For me, this is having sessions where I push myself harder, either as a plan for the session or how I feel that day. If good, then push yourself, and if not, ease back. Keep the variety in your running in ways we discussed earlier, slow distance running most days, interspersed with fartlek, tempo, or interval, or however you wish to experiment.

Do the same in your life. Watch the amount of time you spend on one aspect of your life. Work, family time, personal time, interests and hobbies, volunteering, and of course running. It takes as much dedication to be a good parent or friend as being consistent in your running. Make sure you go out of your way to keep your relationships strong and refreshed. You'll find discipline in your running quickly extends to other areas of your life.

Surprise those important in your life with unexpected gifts or communications. A card thanking somebody for being such a good friend goes a long way to staying in touch even if life is hectic for you. These days you can do this by email or a social media chat. It's never been easier to keep in contact. Don't let your relationships get stale or burn out—they're much more critical than your running and keep you mentally healthy as well.

8. Fuel for Your Body:

Being able to run requires you to maintain a well-oiled machine of body and mind. The mere act of being able to put one foot down after another in rapid succession for any distance is a feat in itself. To do this for many miles each week requires consistently pumping good fuel into your body—healthy and nutritious food. Lack of attention in this area and your body will eventually break down, and you'll end up in the human body shop for major and ongoing renovations.

We all know what healthy food and drink are regarding what's good for our body and what we should avoid. Consuming healthy food also keeps inflammation down in our body, which can be a leading cause of injuries and illness. There's enough information freely available today that there's no excuse to be ignorant of what should go in your mouth and what should be avoided or limited. Be educated and informed when it comes to what is good fuel for your body.

Your doctor may prescribe supplements as you get older. Because of the physics of your body and genes, you may also need to take prescribed medications regardless of adherence to a healthy diet. There are, however, several conditions requiring medicines that can be avoided with just a healthy, consistent diet. It may take time to recover, but by working with your doctor/nutritionist, you can set realistic goals for your running and health conditions.

As with a good diet of food, a feast of positive thoughts helps promote excellent health and is especially conducive for your happiness and enjoyment of life. A daily buffet of negative thoughts is a recipe for unhappiness.

Let your enjoyment of running clear out stale thinking and instead welcome the positive energy you get from doing your running. If you've got a history of poor diet, let your change to a healthier diet spill over to a positive diet of thoughts about yourself and your capabilities. Let your running be the catalyst of feeding your mind with healthy thoughts.

9. Mapping Out Your World:

I believe the routes we choose for our running sessions are essential in our enjoyment of running. I'm fortunate that I live in a relatively rural area with many quiet streets from which to choose. I can vary my runs and terrain by choosing between roads, bike paths, and a running track. Important to me in keeping joy in my running is being outdoors and running in terrain that adds to my enjoyment.

I realize this can be a challenge for those living in urban areas. You may need to find parks and recreational areas to avoid busy streets or places with less-than-ideal surroundings. Even in large cities, I've found pockets where nature has taken hold along pathways, woods, and trails. Research and explore your options.

Routes are one thing, but a schedule is the other side of the coin. The trick, in the beginning, is to keep it simple. Unless you're destined for competitive racing or looking to achieve a specific goal, let how your body feels on any particular day dictate your workout content. I've got a target number of miles I want to achieve each week—it doesn't vary much—but equally as important is the number of days I run. I schedule rest days, but if those days need to change due to my life, then I adjust on the fly. In the beginning, have a flexible schedule and focus on putting in time and miles at an easy pace to build a stamina base.

There's nothing wrong with wanting to improve our running performance once we have a solid base in place. Progress can be more miles or just being able to run at a faster pace. If we don't overextend our body before it's ready, our body will adjust if we take it in small steps, and it will perform predictively for us.

Our life will treat us the same if we're gentle with it. Our discipline in running and our approach also support our enjoyment of life. Our gentleness with ourselves and others will also add to our happiness.

If you interpret my appeal to be gentle as not being driven, then you've misheard me. I'm driven about my running and life to be the best I can be for myself and others. I'm also driven about my work—writing this book requires me to be focused and implementing a routine to ensure it gets completed. But I'm not shutting out the rest of my world because of it. I'm still there for everybody in my life and the other commitments I've made.

As I mentioned before, your capabilities and performance improvement for running will come in fits and starts. It will, and should, take time to build a solid foundation when starting. A course of weeks of slow distance running well within your capabilities will be required before moving into fast/speed work. This is a natural progression; otherwise—*burnout!*

Make and stay with good habits—call it a routine if you want. Your running habits set the discipline for good practices in your daily life as well. It's a model for all aspects of your life. If you can have good habits in your running, then you can have good habits in your life. You're not two different people leading separate lives.

10. Keeping Everything in Perspective:

I have a short life formula document of 3 pages, and I make time to read it a few times each week. You've probably been exposed to some variation of it already. It usually comes in the ritual of a morning/daily formula of some sort. I do mine anytime I want, and I don't get overly concerned about when I do it. You shouldn't either, but it's beneficial to have one and review it often.

My formula has three sections: *future, rules, and principles*. It helps me keep everything in my life in perspective. The mere act of penning one requires the gathering of what's important to you in one place. Whether you share it with anybody else is entirely up to you.

My *future* formula piece covers what I want my life to look like in the coming years. You can label it goals if you wish. It can include work, passions, wealth, travel, and interests. It's a high-level map without specific details on how to get there. But it can be whatever you want it to be.

In the *rules* and *principles* sections, I'm more specific. For example, I decided to affirm that my running does not come before my family. My work does not come before my family. My friends don't come before my family. Yes, our dogs are our family as well. I've family in the U.S. and U.K. and will drop whatever I'm doing if they need me. I believe this reflects who I am.

I also feel that being there for my family is supported by my fitness level, which my running supports and helps my health. So, I've verbiage in my formula covering my running and long-term goals for it.

You can also look at family as what people call today extended family. If you volunteer, then you likely have "*family*" among the people with whom you work. There can be many definitions of the term "*family*."

If running is joy, then so should be the rest of your life. You should celebrate those who bring joy into your life. These can come from anywhere, family and friends, pets or colleagues at work, or with whom you share interests or volunteering.

My point here, as in all this book, is there's a way to take the spirit of your joy for running into your life. It doesn't matter what your age is or at what level your fitness is at; it'll help you achieve a healthy body and mind and make your journey on earth more fulfilling in your pursuit of happiness. Happiness takes work. There isn't a pill for it. It just doesn't fall onto your breakfast plate each day to consume. You don't get it by reading a *"feel good"* book. It starts with you. You can't make anybody else happy in your life before you are. And an excellent place to start is with your running.

In the next and final chapter, it's time for you to run. And if you need some motivation and reasons to get started, then I'll provide them for you. I'll share some of my false starts and how to avoid them. It's a short read.

Get set…

CHAPTER FIFTEEN

Get Set... Go!

"A pessimist sees the difficulty in every opportunity.
An optimist sees the opportunity in every difficulty."
— Winston Churchill

I n England, where I grew up, there were three commands to start a race on the track.

1. On your marks. 2. Get set... (*move to your starting position*) 3. GO! (*explode out of your blocks if you've got them!*).

Well, you've made it through to steps 2 and 3. Everything that came before was preparation for now. These steps are small and quick. If you haven't already started to run, and I strongly suspect you've been running for a while now, reading provides learning, but only action provides experience, then it's time to put this book down and make the decision to run or not to run.

The journey of 2,876 miles begins with the first step. Bruce Tulloh, a famous English distance runner, ran this distance from L.A. to New York in 1965. It took him 65 days, and it was a record for the fastest crossing at the time. But before he took a single running step, he prepared. You could say his decades of running prepared him for such a feat—do the math yourself, he averaged just over 44 miles per day on his coast-to-coast run. Some weeks I'm happy with that as my total!

He wrote a book about his journey across America titled *"Four Million Footsteps."* But it isn't a story just about running. Those 65 days were packed with many adventures, mishaps, and meeting new friends and experiences. Running was the vehicle that provided him the opportunity to make a journey to be remembered. He didn't have any idea what to expect outside his running.

He had a small support team to make it all work. He had a plan and a schedule, and he mostly kept to it. But he also had days when things didn't go as planned. When his body broke down, and he couldn't run. When he had to rest and be flexible, despite the pressure of going for a record. He saw America from the outdoors, and for a brief time, he was part of the landscape. A true traveler across the country with the time to experience and enjoy America in the last days of the 1960s.

I hope you find running helps you through your journeys and provides positive lessons that permeate into all aspects of your life. Lessons about enjoyment and discipline and consistency, and the benefits of good habits.

It starts with running. The rest will come.

Start with the first steps. There doesn't even need to be an investment in any equipment for your first run. If you're not sure if running is for you, pick up your current sneakers you use to walk about the house or do chores, slip on a top and sweats, and go out running for 10 minutes or even 5 minutes.

Talk to your doctor, if necessary, before starting. Discuss it with your family. Start walking if you've never run or have a condition where you need to start slowly. If your first weeks or months are inconsistent and you need to take breaks or rest days, that's okay.

I ran for many years and then stopped; then I started again and stopped. And then again. Each time it took me a while to get restarted. My current running period started about ten years ago. Even during this decade, I've had stages when running 3 miles an hour for 30 minutes was challenging for me both physically and mentally. I had a lot going on in my life at that time, but running was a companion, and it was just to get out and enjoy the activity and not worry much about the pace. To get from one block to the next was often just the goal to complete the run.

Running is a decision, just like life. But it isn't just about running and then leaving it when you take your shoes off. It can bring hope and insight into your life. You start to notice things more around you. Use running to help bring clarity to your life. It's not an exercise of just putting one foot in front of another. It's about forward motion. It's about trying new routines and schedules and looking to keep the interest alive. A time to enjoy exercise and being outdoors.

You'll be excited putting on your running shoes and getting ready for your first or next run.

You can use it to take the stress out of your life. To put on hold, or see clearer, whatever challenges you may be facing that day. I can only imagine what's going on in your life at the moment. I hope all is well. But you may be dealing with grief, or other loss, a complicated family or relationship situation. You may have what you consider a dull or lackluster life and looking to make significant changes to make it better for yourself and those close to you.

I'm not naïve enough to think running can solve all ills, but I've found it's helped and supported me to get through many of my own. Having a pillar such as running gives you the strength to help you face challenges. Life can be complicated and messy at times, and an activity that provides a sanctuary can help us confront and find a path through the turmoil.

My point here, as in all this book, is there's a way to take the spirit of your joy for running into your life. It doesn't matter what your age is or at what level your fitness is at; it'll help you achieve a healthy body and mind and make your journey on earth more fulfilling in your pursuit of happiness.

I hope I've instilled in you a different perspective of running. One that takes it down to its bare essence of fun and enjoyment and removes the competitiveness, eliteness, and science out of it, to leave you with just the play.

It's winter and dark where I am. My run today will begin in about an hour. For the first mile, I'll get the adrenaline pumping just like you'll do when you go out. It's an adventure I invite you to join me in and experience. It happens every time I go out to run and get going. The first mile may be cold or have some stiffness, but I'll protect myself and soon just let the automatic actions of my body and habit take over.

Maybe today will be your first run for exercise ever or since high school. Or it may be your thousandth mile or more. It doesn't matter. We're all at a different stage in our journey, both in running and life. But then, we are, in many respects, all the same.

This may be the last chapter in this book, but it's the beginning of the rest of your life.

What say you?

Are you ready to embrace the opportunity to run? Are you prepared to begin to enjoy running and let it help you also enjoy your life?

Let's begin… GO!

TERMS AND ADDITIONAL MATERIAL

I use several terms in the book that benefit from further context, clarity, and explanation. As many reading this are not yet hard-core runners, I've taken some liberties with terms in the book to simplify options for you, but you're welcome to argue my definitions with other runners over a glass of your favorite beverage. What you call your workouts is entirely up to you.

Similarly, there's some additional material on topics discussed in the book included here for further reference and thought, and information that didn't fit neatly into any of the chapters without taking you off-topic and down rabbit holes.

You can find even more resources at the companion website to this book here: www.RunToEnjoyLife.com

Aerobic and Anaerobic Workouts:

You must understand these two terms and how they differ without you having to read a scientific thesis about your body. Aerobic exercise provides you stamina built up over time by performing slow long-distance running. Aerobic training increases the efficiency of your cardiovascular system so you can pump more oxygen efficiently to your leg muscles to keep them moving over long distances. Aerobic conditioning will lower your resting heart rate—Beats Per Minute (BPM)—over time, as a measure of this efficiency.

Anaerobic workouts involve short bursts of intensive activity and are repeated to provide racing fitness. Anaerobic workouts consist of speed or hill training or both. Examples for running include fast pace over short distances—not just sprinting—but includes 400 – 1-mile intervals and fast hill running. The difference from aerobic training is in anaerobic; the body can't get enough oxygen to the muscles to generate the energy needed, so it obtains energy through its glucose stores, and this quickly leads to a buildup of lactic acid in the muscles, which leads to muscle cramps, pain, and fatigue.

If you want to improve your times and performance, a mixture of both types of workouts in your schedule is needed. Simply put, aerobic workouts provide an ongoing foundation of stamina, and anaerobic can increase speed, particularly over short distances. Most people out to just enjoy their running and get fit will focus on aerobic easy pace workouts.

Interval/Fartlek/Tempo Training:

Interval training is a type of workout where you alternate between slow and fast running. It's also known as High-intensity Interval Training (HIT). Similar to Interval Training is Fartlek workouts. Both these were developed in Europe during the 1930s. Coaches tend to use the term intervals for a workout involving short bursts of a minute or less of speedrunning and more extended periods of rest or slow jogging pace. The intensity can be increased by reducing the rest time between the short bursts. Fartlek tends to be continuous running with alternates of a fast pace for a few miles with an easy pace for the same or longer periods. Both these types of training are classed as anaerobic rather than aerobic.

I've also seen the term interval training used in the context of repetitions over short distances with a rest in between. Emil

Zatopek—the great Czech runner—was reported as running 40-60 fast 400-meter splits on the track in some of his workouts. To save your head spinning, this is an intense workout for 10-15 miles.

I use the term interval/fartlek training in this book, but I don't personally do sprint workouts. Most of my interval training involves fast pace for ½ mile, ¾ mile, or even 1-mile repeats with a slow jog of ¼ to ½ mile between each depending on the repeat distance. I've found they provide an intense workout and help develop better sustainable speed for longer races of 5K and 10K. Additionally, it breaks the monotony of long easy pace runs and adds a sense of play to my running.

You'll also come across the term Tempo training, and this is a workout of long duration—30-40 minutes—at a pace you can sustain for an hour. It's easy to run faster for longer than you should when doing Tempo training, so be careful. It shouldn't feel like you've been in a race when finished.

Sports Science Training:

While not a term mentioned in the book, *Sports Science* aims at understanding what makes elite athletes and informs us in a way that can help us improve our performance. Keeping athletes up to date with current training techniques and preparation can help runners modify their endurance and speed performance.

Footwear:

Footwear is a controversial topic. If you talk to 20 runners, you'll get 20 different responses on the type of shoe they prefer. Running shoes come in all shapes and fittings and, of course, price. They range from lightweight for speed training to stability shoes for more support and longer mileage sessions. I prefer support for all my different workouts, so I have one pair with solid foot support.

I could stop there, but there is a school of thought these days about minimalist shoes, which some folks call finger or barefoot shoes. The view is that because these shoes fit around the individual fingers of the feet, they can move more easily when you run. The additional argument of this school is that our body naturally adjusts to the extra shock-absorbing required on the impact of our feet when running, so the need for built-up shoes containing extra cushioning isn't needed. Given my age and the state of my knees, I prefer to play it safe and have shoes with plenty of support. Moving from one type of shoe to another is better done gradually to avoid injury.

The Marathon:

The marathon isn't a competitive race, at least for most people who enter one. The only competitiveness about it for these folks is with themselves. The goal is to get to the finish line. It was once described to me as more of an adventure than a race. Now I've done a few; yeah, it is.

There are, of course, elite runners where it's a *race* to finish in a qualifying time or a position to get selected for another marathon or team. For these runners, the race can include tactics and even occasionally a tight finish. But this isn't me, nor I suspect the bulk of the people reading this book. For the rest of us, it's a battle with ourselves. And we hope we have prepared well.

Providing you've done the proper preparation, then most people can finish a marathon. There are many books available about training and preparing for a marathon. You can search the Internet and find lots of free and paid advice about schedules and preparation. I've had my wrestles with the distance over the years, and it's a mental game as much as a physical one.

Once you get beyond 20 miles, the marathon will uncover and lay bare any flaw in your preparation, earlier pace, or fluid and energy intake. The initial half of the event is the first 20 miles, and the second half is the final six miles and 385 yards. There is something about the human body that enters fatigue status beyond the 20-mile run. The ultra-marathon distances are beyond the scope of my body at the moment.

Lydiard and Cerutty Influences:

Each generation has its athletic heroes. Mine was no different and was influenced by the success of the middle-distance runners from Europe, New Zealand, and Australia. Two coaching giants of antipodean runners were Arthur Lydiard and Percy Cerutty. It's purported they only met once, and there seemed to be mutual respect between the two. They certainly shared common views around high weekly mileage for endurance building, benefits of hill running, and elements of style. But their personalities were poles apart.

Lydiard took up coaching posts for Mexico and Finland, far from his native New Zealand, and lectured worldwide. Bill Bowerman—the American Track and Field Coach—liaised with Lydiard during his formative coaching years and adopted and modified Lydiard's teachings into his schedules for his athletes in the U.S. Lydiard had a wider influence than Cerutty as his success at the 1960 and 1964 Olympics with his athletes made him highly sought after from countries wishing to develop their athletes for track and field glory.

Percy Cerutty outside his native Australia remained best known for coaching Herb Elliott, although he could include John Landy, Albie Thomas, Betty Cuthbert, and Dave Power in his camp. Unlike Lydiard, he was considered too extreme for many, including philosophical views that went well outside the sphere of influencing just his athletes' running. He focused on technique and hill training less on mechanical, repetitive intervals, such as rival coach Franz Stampfl.

Both Lydiard and Cerutty were giants in their own right and continue to influence today's athletes with their pioneering work finding its way into modified training curriculums for everyday runners.

BIBLIOGRAPHY

I've read many books on different topics. Over the decades, I've absorbed the words of many related to running. I enjoy reading, but like most, I've got my favorites that have influenced me more than others. The list below I've found helpful in shaping some of my thoughts on running, some of them I also specifically re-read for this book.

I've provided a short personal review of each book, but you should not let this determine whether you read it or not. My formative years and role models will be different than yours, and I intend to provide insight into what to expect merely. Something that doesn't resonate with me may well be life-changing for you, and vice versa. After all, it would be a boring world if we all liked the same food and films, and... *books*.

While I've enjoyed reading biographies about champions and Olympic athletes, I've found more practical help for my running in reading about their coaches and how they formulated their ideas and systems. But my reading, and the premise of this book, aren't confined to just running, and so you'll find a few non-related running books helpful in expanding my insights into the larger picture of life.

In the ensuing decades since I started running, we've begun to understand why runners enjoy running. We've sensed the rhythm and flow of it was therapeutic, but we didn't realize just how therapeutic it was in the early days. Today, the benefits touch and help people who are not only looking for health and fitness but ways of dealing with stress, depression, anxiety, and other mental health challenges. Running is benefitting so many people today to deal and cope with their lives beyond keeping fit. I hope you find your answers and help to whatever questions you seek in this book and the shortlist below.

For a complete and additional material, then check out the resources at the companion website for this book at www.RunToEnjoyLife.com

The Joy of Running – *Thaddeus Kostrubala, MD:*

Dr. Kostrubala was a psychiatrist who took up running to get in shape but found it provided a high fitness level for him and a new lease on life. Initially published in 1975 and updated a few times, it chronicles the doctor's experience in his transformation and how he used it to help others. While the book shares aspects of metabolic factors and covers Target Heart Rate (THR) as an element of assisting with training, it isn't a book about the scientific aspects of running.

Running is My Therapy – *Scott Douglas:*

Scott has put together a book of substance around running and its use to cope with stress, anxiety, and depression. Taking his case and detailing much research, he presents examples and lessons of how people have used running to process thoughts differently and help them manage their diagnosis. But he also has plenty of advice for those just wanting to run because they enjoy it.

Spark: The Revolutionary New Science of Exercise and the Brain – *John J. Ratey, MD*

Dr. Ratey is a psychiatrist who has studied and documented the positive impact of exercise on his patients and others. The book explores the science behind why and how exercising can replace or combine with prescription drugs as a treatment for several mental health issues. Although not limited to running as the exercise of choice, if you've been running for any length of time, you'll connect with his descriptions of why it helps. It's one of the rare books I've read that provides the science and explanations to support much of my intuitive feelings on how exercise has helped me cope with life's daily stress and anxiety. An important read.

The Unforgiving Minute – *Ron Clarke:*

Ron Clarke set the world alight in the 1960s with a string of world records over distance running. Clark dominated the period, and though he never won an Olympic Gold medal, he's the name that crops up on every runners' lips who lived through his era as one the greatest over the 5K/10K and 3/6-mile distances. This is his story and details all his major races and thoughts around the training and racing of a remarkable runner in his formative and record-setting years.

Be Fit or Be Damned! – *Percy Cerutty:*

Percy Cerutty was either a genius or a crackpot, depending on which side of the dividing line you place his thoughts. Love him or hate him; you couldn't ignore him. Always controversial as a coach, this book goes way beyond running and exercising and is more of a manifesto on living your life. For me, it's not the most accessible of his books with a jarring writing style but does provide a window into the sanctity in which he held the body and fitness and demanded of those he coached.

Why Die? The Extraordinary Percy Cerutty – *Graem Sims:*

This biography of the controversial man who passed away in 1975, penned by Australian writer Graem Sims is a compelling account of the enigma of *"Percie."* Cerutty was as much a showman as a coach, and this irked and isolated him from the Australian Athletic administrations and eventually from some of the athletes he coached. Percy's style was unconventional and less about dictating personal training schedules and more about lifestyle, mentoring, and technique, expecting his charges to set their schedules and race tactics. Best remembered for coaching Herb Elliott and his Portsea training camp in the dunes south of Melbourne, this book captures the life and spirit of an uncompromising man who was happiest running, teaching, and writing.

Running & Being – *Dr. George Sheehan:*

A book that's a break from traditional running books that are biographies or training manuals. It's a series of articles grouped into topics, where Dr. Sheehan shares his musings and philosophies about running and life. While I can't relate to many of his personal views on running, that didn't stop my enjoyment of the read, and it's by being open-minded; we grow, and he certainly forces you to consider a broader vision for your running.

Running To The Top – *Arthur Lydiard:*

If you're looking for Lydiard's first book, *"Run To The Top,"* published in the 1960s, this isn't it, and that book is now out of print anyway. The content is all about training and schedules and largely ignores Lydiard's history and impact on New Zealand and World middle- and long-distance running scenes. However, this is an excellent resource for any runner who wants to improve their running and understand the *"why"* of training and the use of different workouts and schedules over middle and long distances, including the marathon.

Arthur Lydiard Master Coach – *Garth Gilmour:*

If *"Running To The Top"* introduces Lydiard's training methods focused on aerobic and anaerobic workouts and schedules, then this is his biography, focused on how he developed his philosophies of training athletes. It also journals his ups and downs as a coach as he travels the world, imparting his knowledge to other coaches and athletes in other sports. The story of a remarkable coach and the formulation of his running philosophies developed in the 1950s and '60s and how he made training 100 miles or more a week common in running circles.

Four Million Footsteps – *Bruce Tulloh:*

I read this book shortly after it was first published in 1970. It's currently out of print. But you'd never know in these days of print on demand; maybe we'll see it for sale for an affordable price again. It chronicles his run across America in record-breaking days. One of Britain's elite runners at the end of his elite competitive racing days, he set out on a fascinating journey and set down his experiences and insights on not only running across a continent but through America in the late sixties.

No Bugles No Drums – *Garth Gilmour:*

This is *Peter Snell's* biography – perhaps, along with *Murray Halberg*, the most famous and prolific of Arthur Lydiard's stable of athletes. Snell won three Olympic Gold Medals during the '60s and captured World Records over the ½ and 1 mile and metric equivalents. The read is interesting because it progresses through the maturity of Snell, not only as an athlete but as a person, and how he comes to appreciate the International community of runners. He comes across in the early years as a little provincial and critical of athletes outside the Lydiard camp but then grows to appreciate the International athletic camaraderie of the European and American scenes and becomes his own person outside Lydiard's influence.

Creator – *Steve Chandler:*

If you don't consider yourself a *"creative"* individual, be prepared to overturn that feeling! Steve takes you through his journey to rediscover his creative veins. Witty and entertaining but thought-provoking for anybody who feels when they were dishing out *"creativity,"* they were absent, goofing off and enjoying themselves.

The Enlightened Gardener – *Sydney Banks*:

What's a philosophy book doing in a list of running books? It was written as a parable; it introduced me to the *"three principles"* concepts around how our thoughts and feelings and mind operate and how life works from inside to out. Throughout this book, I allude to how joy in our running can help us enjoy our life, and this provides an articulate read around the mechanics of how to think through these concepts and the implications for you.

You're Invited to Check Out
the Companion Website at:
www.RunToEnjoyLife.com

Throughout this book, I've made references to a companion website. On a topic like running, there are new and revised products and books becoming available monthly. To include specifics in a book becomes futile, and it gets stale and outdated quickly.

Additionally, a growing number of people like to participate in a community that comes together over a topic such as running and what this means to them. Sharing thoughts, opinions, and articles provide a rich resource for "*continuing the conversation,*" so to speak.

So, the website is created for you.

Initially, it will be populated with content of my choosing as it has to start somewhere. But I hope that it will turn more into content added and generated by its users with some moderating to ensure we are inclusive of all opinions in a respectful tone.

You can email me suggestions for enhancements and improvements at cliff@runtoenjoylife.com

Cliff Calderwood

PLEASE REVIEW THIS BOOK

Thank you for purchasing this book and reading it. I hope you will take just a few minutes and leave a review of it. This will help others decide if it is a book for them to enjoy.

If you do it now, that would be best, as life has a way of overtaking us, and we just never get around to doing everything we promise we will do later.

I don't care where you leave the review, although most folks these days tend to leave them at Amazon.

Made in the USA
Middletown, DE
09 October 2021

49609075R00092